Evidence Report/Technology Assessment

Number 135

Management of Eating Disorders

Prepared for:
Agency for Healthcare Research and Quality
U.S. Department of Health and Human Services
540 Gaither Road
Rockville, MD 20850
www.ahrq.gov

Contract No. 290-02-0016

Prepared by:
RTI-UNC Evidence-Based Practice Center, Research Triangle Park, NC

Investigators
Nancy D. Berkman, Ph.D.
Cynthia M. Bulik, Ph.D.
Kimberly A. Brownley, Ph.D.
Kathleen N. Lohr, Ph.D.
Jan A. Sedway, Ph.D.
Adrienne Rooks, B.A.
Gerald Gartlehner, M.D.

AHRQ Publication No. 06-E010
April 2006

Suggested Citation:
Berkman ND, Bulik CM, Brownley KA, Lohr KN, Sedway JA, Rooks A, Gartlehner G. Management of Eating Disorders. Evidence Report/Technology Assessment No. 135. (Prepared by the RTI International-University of North Carolina Evidence-Based Practice Center under Contract No. 290-02-0016.) AHRQ Publication No. 06-E010. Rockville, MD: Agency for Healthcare Research and Quality. April 2006.

Preface

The Agency for Healthcare Research and Quality (AHRQ), through its Evidence-Based Practice Centers (EPCs), sponsors the development of evidence reports and technology assessments to assist public- and private-sector organizations in their efforts to improve the quality of health care in the United States. The report topic was nominated by the American Psychiatric Association (APA) and the Laureate Psychiatric Clinic and Hospital. Funding for this report was provided by the Office of Research on Women's Health at the National Institutes of Health (NIH) and the Health Resources and Services Administration. The reports and assessments provide organizations with comprehensive, science-based information on common, costly medical conditions and new health care technologies. The EPCs systematically review the relevant scientific literature on topics assigned to them by AHRQ and conduct additional analyses when appropriate prior to developing their reports and assessments.

To bring the broadest range of experts into the development of evidence reports and health technology assessments, AHRQ encourages the EPCs to form partnerships and enter into collaborations with other medical and research organizations. The EPCs work with these partner organizations to ensure that the evidence reports and technology assessments they produce will become building blocks for health care quality improvement projects throughout the Nation. The reports undergo peer review prior to their release.

AHRQ expects that the EPC evidence reports and technology assessments will inform individual health plans, providers, and purchasers as well as the health care system as a whole by providing important information to help improve health care quality.

We welcome comments on this evidence report. They may be sent by mail to the Task Order Officer named below at: Agency for Healthcare Research and Quality, 540 Gaither Road, Rockville, MD 20850, or by e-mail to **epc@ahrq.gov.**

Carolyn M. Clancy, M.D.
Director
Agency for Healthcare Research and Quality

Jean Slutsky, P.A., M.S.P.H.
Director, Center for Outcomes and Evidence
Agency for Healthcare Research and Quality

Vivian W. Pinn, M.D.
Director
Office of Research on Women's Health
National Institutes of Health

Beth A. Collins Sharp, R.N., Ph.D.
Acting Director, EPC Program
Agency for Healthcare Research and Quality

Sabrina A. Matoff-Stepp, M.A.
Director
Office of Women's Health
Health Resources and Services Administration

Marian James, Ph.D.
EPC Program Task Order Officer
Agency for Healthcare Research and Quality

Structured Abstract

Objectives. The RTI International—University of North Carolina at Chapel Hill Evidence-based Practice Center (RTI-UNC EPC) systematically reviewed evidence on efficacy of treatment for anorexia nervosa (AN), bulimia nervosa (BN), and binge eating disorder (BED), harms associated with treatments, factors associated with the treatment efficacy and with outcomes of these conditions, and whether treatment and outcomes for these conditions differ by sociodemographic characteristics.

Data Sources. We searched MEDLINE®, the Cumulative Index to Nursing and Applied Health (CINAHL), PSYCHINFO, the Educational Resources Information Center (ERIC), the National Agricultural Library (AGRICOLA), and Cochrane Collaboration libraries.

Review Methods. We reviewed each study against a priori inclusion/exclusion criteria. For included articles, a primary reviewer abstracted data directly into evidence tables; a second senior reviewer confirmed accuracy. We included studies published from 1980 to September, 2005, in all languages. Studies had to involve populations diagnosed primarily with AN, BN, or BED and report on eating, psychiatric or psychological, or biomarker outcomes.

Results. We report on 30 treatment studies for AN, 47 for BN, 25 for BED, and 34 outcome studies for AN, 13 for BN, 7 addressing both AN and BN, and 3 for BED.

The AN literature on medications was sparse and inconclusive. Some forms of family therapy are efficacious in treating adolescents. Cognitive behavioral therapy (CBT) may reduce relapse risk for adults after weight restoration.

For BN, fluoxetine (60 mg/day) reduces core bulimic symptoms (binge eating and purging) and associated psychological features in the short term. Individual or group CBT decreases core behavioral symptoms and psychological features in both the short and long term. How best to treat individuals who do not respond to CBT or fluoxetine remains unknown.

In BED, individual or group CBT reduces binge eating and improves abstinence rates for up to 4 months after treatment; however, CBT is not associated with weight loss. Medications may play a role in treating BED patients. Further research addressing how best to achieve both abstinence from binge eating and weight loss in overweight patients is needed.

Higher levels of depression and compulsivity were associated with poorer outcomes in AN; higher mortality was associated with concurrent alcohol and substance use disorders. Only depression was consistently associated with poorer outcomes in BN; BN was not associated with an increased risk of death. Because of sparse data, we could reach no conclusions concerning BED outcomes.

No or only weak evidence addresses treatment or outcomes difference for these disorders.

Conclusions. The literature regarding treatment efficacy and outcomes for AN, BN, and BED is of highly variable quality. In future studies, researchers must attend to issues of statistical power, research design, standardized outcome measures, and sophistication and appropriateness of statistical methodology.

Contents

Figures

Tables

Appendixes

Appendix A: Exact Search Strings
Appendix B: Sample Data Collection Forms
Appendix C: Evidence Tables
Appendix D: List of Excluded Articles
Appendix E: Acknowledgments

Appendixes and Evidence Tables for this report are provided electronically at
http://www.ahrq.gov/downloads/pub/evidence/pdf/eatingdisorders/eatdis.pdf.

Executive Summary

Introduction

The RTI International–University of North Carolina at Chapel Hill Evidence-based Practice Center (RTI-UNC EPC) conducted a systematic review of the literature on key questions concerning anorexia nervosa (AN), bulimia nervosa (BN), and eating disorders not otherwise specified (EDNOS) (focusing on binge eating disorder [BED]) to address questions posed by the American Psychiatric Association and Laureate Psychiatric Hospital through the Agency for Healthcare Research and Quality (AHRQ). Funding was provided by AHRQ, the Office of Research on Women's Health at the National Institutes of Health, and the Health Resources and Services Administration. We received guidance and input from a Technical Expert Panel (TEP).

We systematically reviewed the evidence on two categories of issues—treatment and outcomes for AN, BN, and BED—in six key questions (KQs): (1) efficacy of treatment, (2) harms associated with treatment, (3) factors associated with the efficacy of treatment, (4) whether efficacy of treatment differs by sex, gender, age, race, ethnicity, or cultural group, (5) factors associated with outcomes, and (6) whether outcomes differ by sex, gender, age, race, ethnicity, or cultural group.

AN is marked by low body weight, fear of weight gain, disturbance in the way in which one's body size is perceived, denial of illness, or undue influence of weight on self-evaluation. Although amenorrhea is a diagnostic criterion, it is of questionable relevance.

BN is characterized by recurrent episodes of binge eating in combination with some form of compensatory behavior. Binge eating is the consumption of an uncharacteristically large amount of food by social comparison coupled with a feeling of being out of control. Compensatory behaviors include self-induced vomiting; misuse of laxatives, diuretics, or other agents; fasting; and excessive exercise.

BED is marked by binge eating in the absence of compensatory behaviors, a series of associated features of binge eating, and marked distress regarding binge eating. Overweight and obesity are commonly seen in individuals with BED.

Although rigorous epidemiologic data are lacking in the United States, the mean prevalence of AN is 0.3 percent, of subthreshold AN 0.37 percent to 1.3 percent, of BN 1.0 percent, and of BED 0.7 percent to 3.0 percent. Mortality from AN is about 5 percent per decade of followup. Treatment for severe AN can involve inpatient or partial hospitalization in costly specialized settings. Inadequate insurance coverage often truncates the recommended duration of treatment. Treatment costs for AN are higher than those for obsessive-compulsive disorder and comparable to those for schizophrenia. In contrast, treatment for BN in the United States is typically on an outpatient basis.

Methods

We searched MEDLINE®, the Cumulative Index to Nursing and Applied Health (CINAHL), PSYCHINFO, the Educational Resources Information Center (ERIC), the National Agricultural Library (AGRICOLA), and Cochrane Collaboration libraries. Based on key questions and discussion with our TEP, we generated a list of article inclusion and exclusion criteria. We reviewed studies of humans, ages 10 years and older, of both sexes, published in all languages and from all nations, from 1980 to September 2005. Studies had to include populations diagnosed primarily with AN, BN, or BED and to report on at least one of our outcomes

1

and from all nations, from 1980 to September 2005. Studies had to include populations diagnosed primarily with AN, BN, or BED and to report on at least one of our outcomes categories of interest: eating-related behaviors, psychiatric and psychological outcomes, and biomarker measures. We reviewed each abstract and article systematically against a priori criteria to determine whether to include it in the review. One reviewer initially evaluated abstracts for inclusion or exclusion. If that reviewer concluded that the article should be included in the review, it was retained. Articles that the reviewer determined did not meet our criteria were re-reviewed by a senior reviewer who could include the article if she disagreed with the initial determination. We assigned each excluded article a reason for exclusion.

The RTI-UNC EPC team abstracted data from included articles directly into evidence tables. For both the treatment and the outcomes literatures, a primary reviewer abstracted data directly into evidence tables; a second (senior) reviewer confirmed accuracy, completeness, and consistency. The two staff reconciled all disagreements about information in evidence tables.

Each abstractor independently evaluated study quality. Because of differences in the treatment and outcomes literature, we evaluated the two bodies of literature using separate criteria. For the treatment literature, our evaluation used 25 items in 11 categories: (1) research aim/study question, (2) study population, (3) randomization, (4) blinding, (5) interventions, (6) outcomes, (7) statistical analysis, (8) results, (9) discussion, (10) external validity, and (11) funding/sponsorship. For the outcomes literature, we evaluated the evidence against 17 items in 8 categories: (1) research aim/study question, (2) study population, (3) eating disorder diagnosis method, (4) study design, (5) statistical analysis, (6) results/outcome measurement, (7) external validity, and (8) discussion.

We focused our analysis on studies that received fair or good quality ratings. This included 19 studies discussed in 22 articles concerning treatment for AN: 38 studies discussed in 48 articles concerning treatment for BN: 20 studies discussed in 21 articles concerning treatment for BED: 26 studies discussed in 32 articles concerning outcomes for AN: 9 studies discussed in 13 articles concerning outcomes for BN: 7 studies discussed in 7 articles concerning outcomes for both AN and BN: and 3 studies discussed in 3 articles concerning outcomes for BED.

Results

Treatment Studies

Anorexia Nervosa. We divided the treatment literature into medication-only (generally in the context of clinical management or hospitalization), medication plus behavioral intervention, and behavioral intervention only for either adults or adolescents. The literature regarding medication treatments for AN is sparse and inconclusive. The vast majority of studies had small sample sizes and rarely had adequate statistical power to allow for definitive conclusions. Although studies did include medication administered during or after inpatient intervention, no AN studies that systematically combined medication with behavioral interventions met our inclusion criteria, revealing a substantial gap in the literature.

In the behavioral intervention literature, preliminary evidence suggests that cognitive behavioral therapy (CBT) may reduce relapse risk for adults with AN after weight restoration. Sufficient evidence does not exist to determine whether CBT has any effect during the acute phase of the illness, and one study, also requiring replication, showed that a manual-based treatment combining elements of sound clinical management and supportive psychotherapy by a specialist was more effective than CBT during the acute phase. Family therapy as currently conceptualized does not appear to be effective with adults with AN with longer duration of illness. Specific forms of family therapy initially focusing on parental control of renutrition is efficacious in treating AN in adolescents and leads to clinically meaningful weight gain and psychological change. The lack of follow-up data compromises our ability to determine the extent to which treatment gains are maintained.

Bulimia Nervosa. In medication trials, fluoxetine (60 mg/day) administered for 6 weeks to 18 weeks reduced the core bulimia symptoms of binge eating and purging and associated psychological features in the short term. The 60 mg dose performs better than lower doses and is associated with prevention of relapse at 1 year. Evidence for the long-term effectiveness of relatively brief medication treatment does not exist. The optimal duration of treatment and the optimal strategy for maintenance of treatment gains are unknown.

Studies that combine drugs and behavioral interventions provide only preliminary evidence regarding the optimal combination of medication and psychotherapy or self-help. How best to treat individuals who do not respond to CBT or fluoxetine remains a major shortcoming of the literature. For behavioral interventions for BN, CBT administered individually or in group format is effective in reducing the core behavioral symptoms of binge eating and purging and psychological features in both the short and long term. Further evidence is required to establish the role for self-help in reducing bulimic behaviors.

Binge Eating Disorder. For BED, we addressed two critical outcomes—decrease in binge eating and decrease in weight in overweight individuals. Various medications were studied, including selective serotonin reuptake inhibitors (SSRIs); a combined serotonin, dopamine, and norepinephrine uptake inhibitor; tricyclic antidepressants; an anticonvulsant; and one appetite suppressant. In short-term trials, SSRIs led to greater rates of reduction in target eating, psychiatric and weight symptoms, and severity of illness than placebo controls. However, in the absence of clear endpoint data, and in the absence of data regarding abstinence from binge eating, we cannot judge the magnitude of the clinical impact of these interventions. Moreover, in the absence of follow-up data after drug discontinuation, we do not know whether observed changes in binge eating, depression, and weight persist.

The combination of CBT plus medication may improve both binge eating and weight loss, although sufficient trials have not been done to determine definitively which medications are best at producing and maintaining weight loss. Moreover, the optimal duration of medication treatment for sustained weight loss has not yet been addressed empirically.

Collectively, clinical trials incorporating CBT for BED indicated that CBT decreases either the number of binge days or the actual number of reported binge episodes. CBT leads to greater rates of abstinence than does a waiting list control approach when administered either individually or in group format, and this abstinence persists for up to 4 months posttreatment. CBT also improves the psychological aspects of BED, such as ratings of restraint, hunger, and disinhibition. Results are mixed as to whether CBT improves self-rated depression in this population. Finally, CBT does not appear to produce decreases in weight.

Various forms of self-help were efficacious in decreasing binge days, binge eating episodes, and psychological features associated with BED. Self-help also led to greater abstinence from binge eating than waiting list; short-term abstinence rates approximate those seen in face-to-face psychotherapy trials.

Strength of Evidence in Treatment Literature. We graded the strength of the body of evidence for each question separately. For efficacy of treatment (KQ 1), we graded evidence for AN treatment as weak, that for BN medication and behavioral interventions as strong, and that for BED therapies as moderate. For harms associated with treatment (KQ 2), we graded medication interventions for BN and BED as consistently strong; the literatures for all AN interventions and all other BN and BED interventions were graded as weak to nonexistent because many studies failed to address harms associated with treatment. For factors associated with efficacy of treatment (KQ 3), with the exception of behavioral interventions for BN, which we graded as moderate, we graded the literature uniformly as weak. No published literature provided evidence on whether the efficacy of treatment for these conditions differs by sociodemographic factors (KQ 4). Overall, the literature on the treatment of AN in particular was deficient.

Outcomes Literature

Outcomes of Eating Disorders. One prospective cohort study, conducted in Sweden, followed individuals with AN in the community. Over a 10-year period, approximately half of the group had fully recovered; a small percentage continued to suffer from AN, and the remainder still had other eating disorders. Members of the AN group no longer differed from those in the comparison group in terms of weight, but they continued to be more depressed and to suffer from a variety of personality disorders, obsessive-compulsive disorder, Asperger syndrome, and autism spectrum disorders.

The remaining AN studies followed patient populations. Typically, at least one-half of the patients no longer suffered from AN at followup. However, many continued to have other eating disorders such as BN or EDNOS, and mortality was significantly higher than would be expected in the population matched by sex and age. Factors associated with recovery or good outcomes included lower levels of depression and compulsivity. Factors associated with increased mortality included concurrent alcohol and substance use disorders.

All of the BN outcomes studies followed patient populations. This literature emphasizes comparisons of various definitions of disease outcomes and diagnostic subtypes. Generally, more than one-half of the patients followed no longer had a BN diagnosis at the end of the study. A substantial percentage continued to suffer from other eating disorders, but BN was not associated with an increased mortality risk. A limited number of analyses uncovered factors significantly associated with outcomes of this disease, but only depression was consistently associated with worse outcomes.

Only sparse evidence addresses factors associated with BED outcomes. The three included studies have vastly different designs and research questions; more importantly, they do not converge on any systematic findings. Recalling that no studies of EDNOS outcomes exist, we conclude that the literature regarding outcomes of both EDNOS in general and BED in particular is seriously lacking; we believe that no conclusions can be drawn about factors influencing outcomes of these disorders.

Age of AN disease onset was examined in several AN outcomes studies. However, the relation between this variable and outcomes was mixed. No additional differences by participant sex, gender, age, race, ethnicity, or cultural group emerged from the AN, BN, or BED outcomes literature.

Strength of Evidence in Outcomes Literature. The strength of the evidence addressing factors associated with outcomes among individuals with AN and BN is moderate. In contrast, given the limited information about factors related to outcomes among individuals with BED (KQ 5), we rated BED evidence as weak. We used the body of literature concerning KQ 5 to examine differences in outcomes by sociodemographic factors (KQ 6). We graded the AN literature as weak and the BN and BED literature as nonexistent.

Discussion

In conclusion, the literature regarding treatment efficacy and outcome for AN, BN, and BED is of highly variable quality. In the treatment literature, the largest deficiency rests with treatment efficacy for AN where the literature was weakest. Future studies require large numbers of participants, multiple sites, appropriate biomarker outcomes, and clear delineation of the age of participants. For BN, future studies should address novel treatments for the disorder, optimal duration of intervention, and optimal approaches for those who do not respond to medication or CBT. For BED, future studies should identify interventions that are effective for both elimination of binge eating and reduction of weight (in overweight individuals), optimal duration of intervention, and effective strategies for prevention of relapse. For all three disorders, exploration of additional treatment approaches is warranted. In addition, for all three disorders, greater attention must be paid to factors influencing outcomes, harms associated with treatment, and differential efficacy by sex, gender, age, race, ethnicity, or cultural group.

For all three disorders, consensus definitions of remission, recovery, and relapse are essential. Greater attention to disease presentations currently grouped under the heading of EDNOS is required for both treatment and outcome literature. For outcome studies, especially for BN and BED, population-based cohort studies with comparison groups and adequate durations of followup are required. For both future treatment and outcome studies, researchers must carefully attend to issues of statistical power, research design including the use of similar outcome measures across studies, and sophistication and appropriateness of statistical analyses.

Evidence Report

Chapter 1. Introduction

Scope of the Problem

The eating disorders discussed in this report include anorexia nervosa (AN), bulimia nervosa (BN), and eating disorders not otherwise specified (EDNOS). Although rigorous epidemiologic data specific only to the United States are lacking, the mean prevalence of AN in young females in Western Europe and the United States is 0.3 percent and the mean prevalence of BN is 1.0 percent. Clinically concerning subthreshold conditions are more prevalent.[1] These eating disorders are associated with substantial morbidity and mortality.[2,3] The financial and social impact of these potentially fatal disorders on disability, productivity, and quality of life remains unknown.

Anorexia Nervosa

Clinical Characteristics

AN is a serious psychiatric illness marked by an inability to maintain a normal healthy body weight, often dropping well below 85 percent of ideal body weight. Patients who are still growing fail to make expected increases in weight (and often height) and bone density. Despite increasing weight loss, individuals with AN continue to obsess about weight, remain dissatisfied with the perceived size of their bodies, and engage in an array of unhealthy behaviors to perpetuate weight loss (e.g., purging, dieting, excessive exercise, fasting). Individuals with AN place central importance on their shape and weight as a marker of self-worth and self-esteem. Although amenorrhea is a diagnostic criterion, it is of questionable relevance. There do not appear to be meaningful differences between individuals with AN who do and do not menstruate.[4,5] Typical personality features of individuals with AN include perfectionism, obsessionality, anxiety, harm avoidance, and low self-esteem.[6]

The most common comorbid psychiatric conditions include major depression[7,8] and anxiety disorders.[9,10] Anxiety disorders often predate the onset of the eating disorder,[9,10] and depression often persists post-recovery.[11]

Diagnostic Criteria

Table 1 presents the diagnostic criteria that authors of articles reviewed in this report use. They include Russell criteria,[12] Feighner criteria,[13] Diagnostic and Statistical Manual for Mental Disorders III, III-R and IV (DSM III, III-R, and IV),[14-16] and the International Classification of Diseases-Versions 9 and 10 (ICD-9 and ICD-10).[17]

Epidemiology

The mean prevalence of AN in young females in Western Europe and the United States is 0.3 percent.[1] The prevalence of subthreshold AN, defined as one criterion short of threshold, is greater—ranging from 0.37 percent to 1.3 percent.[18,19]

Although awareness of the disorder has increased, the data on changing incidence are conflicting. Some studies suggest that the incidence is increasing,[20-26] and others report stable

Table 1. Diagnostic criteria: anorexia nervosa

Diagnostic Criteria	
Russell's Criteria for Anorexia Nervosa	1. Patient resorts to a variety of devices aimed at achieving weight loss (starvation, vomiting, laxatives, etc.) 2. Evidence of an endocrine disorder, amenorrhea in the female, and loss of sexual potency and interest in the male 3. Patient manifests the characteristic psychopathology of a morbid fear of becoming fat. This is accompanied by a distorted judgment by the patient of her body size
Feighner's Criteria for Anorexia Nervosa	1. Onset prior to age 25 2. Anorexia with accompanying weight loss of at least 25 percent of original body weight 3. A distorted implacable attitude toward eating food or weight that overrides hunger, admonitions, reassurances, and threats 4. No known medical illness accounts for the anorexia [nervosa] and weight loss 5. No other known psychiatric disorder, with particular reference to primary affective disorders, schizophrenia, obsessive, and compulsive and phobic neurosis 6. At least two of the following manifestations: amenorrhea, lanugo, bradycardia, periods of overactivity, episodes of bulimia, vomiting
DSM III Criteria for Anorexia Nervosa (307.10)	A. Intense fear of becoming obese, which does not diminish as weight loss progresses B. Disturbance of body image (e.g., claiming to "feel fat" even when emaciated) C. Weight loss of at least 25% of original body weight or, if under 18 years of age, weight loss from original body weight plus projected weight gain expected from growth charts may be combined to make the 25% D. Refusal to maintain body weight over a minimal normal weight for age and height E. No known physical illness that would account for the weight loss
DSM III-R Criteria for Anorexia Nervosa (307.10)	A. Refusal to maintain body weight over a minimal normal weight for age and height (e.g., weight loss leading to maintenance of body weight 15% below that expected or failure to make expected weight gain during period of growth, leading to body weight 15% below that expected) B. Intense fear of gaining weight or becoming fat, even though underweight C. Disturbance in the way in which one's body weight, size, or shape is experienced (e.g., the person claims to "feel fat" even when emaciated, believes that one area of the body is "too fat" even when obviously underweight) D. In females, absence of at least three consecutive menstrual cycles when otherwise expected to occur (primary and secondary amenorrhea). (A woman is considered to have amenorrhea if her periods occur only following hormone, e.g., estrogen, administration.)
DSM IV Criteria for Anorexia Nervosa (307.10)	A. Refusal to maintain body weight at or above a minimally normal weight for age and height (e.g., weight loss leading to maintenance of body weight less than 85% of that expected or failure to make expected weight gain during period of growth, leading to body weight less than 85% of that expected). B. Intense fear of gaining weight or becoming fat, even though underweight. C. Disturbance in the way in which one's body weight or shape is experienced, undue influence of body weight or shape on self-evaluation, or denial of the seriousness of the current low body weight. D. In postmenarchal females, amenorrhea i.e., the absence of at least three consecutive cycles. (A woman is considered to have amenorrhea if her periods occur only following hormone, e.g., estrogen administration.) *Specify type:* • **Restricting Type:** During the current episode of anorexia nervosa, the person has not regularly engaged in binge-eating or purging behavior (i.e., self-induced vomiting or the misuse of laxatives, diuretics, or enemas). • **Binge-Eating/Purging Type:** During the current episode of anorexia nervosa, the person has regularly engaged in binge-eating or purging behavior (i.e., self-induced vomiting or the misuse of laxatives, diuretics, or enemas).

DSM, Diagnostic and Statistical Manual; ICD, International Classification of Diseases.
For citations, see text.

Table 1. Diagnostic criteria: anorexia nervosa (continued)

Diagnostic Criteria	
ICD-9 Criteria for Anorexia Nervosa (307.1)	A disorder in which the main features are persistent active refusal to eat and marked loss of weight
	The level of activity and alertness is characteristically high in relation to the degree of emaciation
	Typically the disorder begins in teenage girls but it may sometimes begin before puberty and rarely occurs in males
	Amenorrhoea is usual and there may be a variety of other changes including slow pulse and respiration and low body temperature and dependent oedema
	Unusual eating habits and attitudes toward food are typical and sometimes starvation follows or alternates with periods of overeating
	The accompanying psychiatric symptoms are diverse
ICD-10 Criteria for Anorexia Nervosa (F50.0)	A. There is weight loss or, in children, a lack of weight gain, leading to a body weight at least 15% below the normal or expected weight for age and height B. The weight loss is self-induced by avoidance of "fattening foods" C. There is self-perception of being too fat, with an intrusive dread of fatness, which leads to a self-imposed low weight threshold D. A widespread endocrine disorder involving the hypothalamic-pituitary-gonadal axis is manifested in women as amenorrhoea and in men as a loss of sexual interest and potency. (An apparent exception is the persistence of vaginal bleeds in anorexic women who are on replacement hormonal therapy, most commonly taken as a contraceptive pill) E. The disorder does not meet criteria A or B for bulimia nervosa
ICD-10 Criteria for Atypical Anorexia Nervosa (F50.1)	Disorder that fulfills some of the features of anorexia nervosa but in which the overall clinical picture does not justify that diagnosis. For instance, one of the key symptoms, such as amenorrhoea or marked dread of being fat, may be absent in the presence of marked weight loss or weight-reducing behavior. This diagnosis should not be made in the presence of known physical disorders associated with weight loss

rates.[27-31] Epidemiological studies indicate that the peak age of onset is between 15 and 19 years.[32] Anecdotal reports suggest increasing presentations in prepubertal children[33] and new onset cases in mid- and late-life.[34,35] The gender ratio for AN is approximately 9:1, women to men.[16]

Etiology

The etiology of AN remains incompletely understood. Although numerous psychological, social, and biological factors have been implicated as potentially causal, few specific risk factors have been consistently replicated in studies of the etiology of the disorder.[36,37] Although not disorder-specific, common risk factors across eating disorders include sex, race or ethnicity, childhood eating and gastrointestinal problems, elevated shape and weight concerns, negative self-evaluation, sexual abuse and other adverse events, and general psychiatric comorbidity.[36] In addition, prematurity, smallness for gestational age, and cephalohematoma have been identified as risk factors for AN.[38]

The preponderance of reports from western cultures fueled early conceptualizations of AN as a culturally determined disorder, but the past decade of biological and genetic research has revealed that AN is familial[39] and that the observed familial aggregation is attributable primarily to genetic factors.[40-42] Moreover, molecular genetic studies have identified areas of the human genome that may harbor susceptibility loci for AN[43,44] and specific genes that may influence risk.[45,46]

In addition, an array of pharmacologic, genetic, and neuroimaging studies have identified fundamental disturbances in serotonergic function in individuals with AN even after recovery.[47] Although serotonin has received considerable research attention, given the interrelatedness of neurotransmitter function, other neurotransmitter systems, most notably dopamine, are also implicated in these disorders.[48] The ultimate understanding of AN etiology will likely include main effects of both biological and environmental factors as well as their interactions and correlations.

Course of Illness

AN has serious medical and psychological consequences that can persist even after recovery. Features associated with the eating disorder including depression, anxiety, social withdrawal, heightened self-consciousness, fatigue, and multiple medical complications.[7,49-51] The social toll of AN interferes with normal adolescent development.[52] Across psychiatric disorders, the highest risks of premature death, from both natural and unnatural causes, are from substance abuse and eating disorders.[53]

A history of AN is associated with greater problems with reproduction,[54] osteoporosis,[55-57] continued low body mass index (BMI, a commonly used measure of normal weight, overweight, or obesity calculated as weight in kilograms divided by height in meters squared [kg/m^2]), and major depression.[11] Chapter 6 reviews eating-related, psychological, and biomarker-measured outcomes of AN in detail.

Treatment

Given the high morbidity and mortality associated with AN, developing effective treatments for AN is critical. Because of the frequent medical complications and nutritional compromise, clinical practice typically includes a comprehensive medical evaluation and nutritional counseling. Typically, less medically compromised cases of AN are treated on an outpatient basis by psychiatrists, psychologists, and other therapists with primary care providers managing medical care. Professional organizations have developed several English-language treatment guidelines or position papers for the treatment of AN; these include the American Psychiatric Association,[58] the National Institute for Clinical Excellence,[59] the Society for Adolescent Medicine,[60] the American Academy of Pediatrics,[61] and the Royal Australian and New Zealand College of Psychiatrists.[62]

Psychotherapeutic approaches include individual psychotherapy (cognitive-behavioral, interpersonal, behavioral, and psychodynamic), family therapy (especially for younger patients), and group therapy. The American Psychiatric Association Working Group on Eating Disorders concluded that hospitalization is appropriate for individuals below 75 percent of ideal body weight.[58] Weight is not the only parameter to be considered in level of care decisions. Other considerations include medical complications, suicide attempt or plan, failure of outpatient or partial hospitalization treatment, psychiatric comorbidity, role impairment, poor psychosocial support, compromised pregnancy, and lack of availability of less intensive treatment options.[58] Such treatment commonly involves highly specialized multidisciplinary teams including psychologists, psychiatrists, internists or pediatricians, nutritionists, social workers, and nurse specialists.

Striegel-Moore et al. reported the average length of stay to be 26 days using an insurance database of approximately 4 million individuals in the United States;[63] this is substantially shorter than the lengths of stay in other countries, including New Zealand (72 days)[64] and Europe, which ranges from 40.6 days (Finland) to 135.8 days (Switzerland).[65] They found that, per patient, AN treatment costs in the United States were higher than those for obsessive-compulsive disorder and comparable to those for schizophrenia, both of which have prevalences similar to those of AN.[63]

A workshop sponsored by the National Institute of Mental Health (NIMH) examined problems in conducting research on AN treatment.[66] It highlighted obstacles such as relatively low incidence and prevalence, lack of consensus on best treatments, variable presentation within the patient population based on age and illness factors, high costs of providing treatment, and the complex interaction of medical and psychiatric problems associated with the illness. This report also highlighted the importance of improving and expanding the workforce in the eating disorders research field.

Bulimia Nervosa

Clinical Characteristics

BN is characterized by recurrent episodes of binge eating in combination with some form of inappropriate compensatory behavior. Binge eating is the consumption of an abnormally large amount of food coupled with a feeling of being out of control. Compensatory behaviors (aimed at preventing weight gain) include self-induced vomiting; the misuse of laxatives, diuretics, or other agents; fasting; and excessive exercise.

The onset of BN usually occurs in adolescence or early adulthood and is most frequently seen in women who are of normal body weight.[16] Although the gender ratio is approximately 9:1, women to men, the diagnostic criteria themselves are gender-biased. In contrast to women, men tend to present with a greater reliance on nonpurging forms of compensatory behavior such as excessive exercise.[67,68] Considerations of differences in the clinical presentation of BN in men may lead to revised estimates.[67,69]

Approximately 80 percent of patients with BN are diagnosed with another psychiatric disorder at some time in their life.[70] Commonly comorbid psychiatric conditions include anxiety disorders, major depression, dysthymia, substance use, and personality disorders.[9,71-77] Personality features of individuals with BN include some features shared with AN such as high harm avoidance, perfectionism, and low self-esteem. Features more specific to BN include higher novelty seeking, higher impulsivity, lower self-directedness, and lower cooperativeness.[78-80]

Diagnostic Criteria

Table 2 presents DSM III, III-R, and IV and ICD-10 diagnostic criteria for BN. According to DSM IV criteria, a diagnosis of BN requires a minimum of 3 months of binge eating and compensatory behavior occurring twice a week or more. Similar to AN, individuals have to report the undue influence of weight and shape on their self-esteem. In addition, BN is diagnosed

Table 2. Diagnostic criteria: bulimia nervosa

Diagnostic Criteria	

DSM III Criteria for Bulimia Nervosa (307.51)	A. Recurrent episodes of binge eating (rapid consumption of a large amount of food in a discrete period of time, usually less than two hours)
	B. At least three of the following:
	  (1) consumption of high-caloric, easily ingested food during a binge
	  (2) inconspicuous eating during a binge
	  (3) termination of such eating episodes by abdominal pain, sleep, social interruption, or self-induced vomiting
	  (4) repeated attempts to lose weight by severely restrictive diets, self-induced vomiting, or use of cathartics or diuretics
	  (5) frequent weight fluctuations greater than 10 pounds due to alternating binges and fasts
	C. Awareness that the eating pattern is abnormal and fear of not being able to stop eating voluntarily
	D. Depressed mood and self-deprecating thoughts following eating binges
	E. The bulimic episodes are not due to anorexia nervosa or any known physical disorder

DSM III-R Criteria for Bulimia Nervosa (307.51)	A. Recurrent episodes of binge eating (rapid consumption of a large amount of food in a discrete period of time) B. A feeling of lack of control over eating behavior during the eating binges C. The person regularly engages in either self-induced vomiting, use of laxatives or diuretics, strict dieting or fasting, or vigorous exercise in order to prevent weight gain D. A minimum average of two binge eating episodes a week for at least 3 months E. Persistent overconcern with body shape and weight

DSM IV Criteria for Bulimia Nervosa (307.51)	A. Recurrent episodes of binge eating. An episode of binge eating is characterized by both of the following:
	  (1) Eating, in a discrete period of time (e.g., within any 2-hour period), an amount of food that is definitely larger than most people would eat during a similar period of time and under similar circumstances
	  (2) A sense of lack of control over eating during the episode (e.g., a feeling that one cannot stop eating or control what or how much one is eating)
	B. Recurrent inappropriate compensatory behavior in order to prevent weight gain, such as self-induced vomiting; misuse of laxatives, diuretics, enemas, or other medications; fasting or excessive exercise
	C. The binge eating and inappropriate compensatory behaviors both occur, on average, at least twice a week for 3 months
	D. Self-evaluation is unduly influenced by body shape and weight
	E. The disturbance does not occur exclusively during episodes of anorexia nervosa
	
	Specify type:
	Purging type: During the current episode of bulimia nervosa, the person has regularly engaged in self-induced vomiting or the misuse of laxatives, diuretics, or enemas
	Nonpurging type: During the current episode of bulimia nervosa, the person has used inappropriate compensatory behaviors, such as fasting or excessive exercise, but has not regularly engaged in self-induced vomiting or the misuse of laxatives, diuretics, or enemas

DSM, Diagnostic and Statistical Manual; ICD, International Classification of Diseases.
For citations, see text.

Table 2. Diagnostic criteria: bulimia nervosa (continued)

Diagnostic Criteria	

ICD-10 Criteria for Bulimia Nervosa (F50.2)	A. There are recurrent episodes of overeating (at least twice a week over a period of 3 months) in which large amounts of food are consumed in short periods of time
	B. There is persistent preoccupation with eating, and a strong desire or sense of compulsion to eat (craving)
	C. The patient attempts to counteract the "fattening" effects of food by one or more of the following:
	  (1) self-induced vomiting
	  (2) self-induced purging
	  (3) alternating periods of starvation
	  (4) use of drugs such as appetite suppressants, thyroid preparations, or diuretics; when bulimia occurs in diabetic patients they may choose to neglect their insulin treatment
	D. There is self-perception of being too fat, with an intrusive dread of fatness (usually leading to underweight)

ICD-10 Criteria for Atypical Bulimia Nervosa (F50.3)	Disorder that fulfills some of the features of bulimia nervosa, but in which the overall clinical picture does not justify that diagnosis. For instance, there may be recurrent bouts of overeating or overuse of purgatives without significant weight change, or the typical overconcern about body shape and weight may be absent

secondary to AN (i.e., the illness is diagnosed as BN only if the criteria for AN are not met). Thus, to be diagnosed with BN, individuals should have a BMI greater than 17.5 or the equivalent in children and adolescents. The DSM distinguishes two subtypes of BN based on the individual's compensatory behavior: purging (including vomiting and misuse of laxatives, diuretics, or enemas) and nonpurging (restricted eating and exercise). The ICD-10[17] describes only the compensatory mechanisms of vomiting and use of purgatives for BN, because of societal pathologizing of vomiting and laxative misuse when compared with exercise or restrictive eating. ICD-10 does acknowledge alternate periods of starvation in BN.

Epidemiology

A recent review estimated the prevalence of BN to be 1 percent for women and 0.1 percent for men across Western Europe and the United States.[1] The prevalence of subthreshold BN was considerably higher: 1.5 percent for full syndrome and 5.4 percent for partial syndrome. Because of the late introduction of BN into psychiatric nomenclature, few studies have explored temporal changes in the incidence of the disorder. Moreover, few studies have estimated the prevalence of BN among children and adolescents.

Etiology

Historically, like AN, BN has been conceptualized as having sociocultural origins. Substantial familial aggregation of BN has been reported.[39] Twin studies reveal a moderate to substantial contribution of additive genetic factors (between 54 percent and 83 percent) and unique environmental factors to BN.[81,82] Linkage analyses have identified areas on chromosome 10p that may be implicated in BN.[83] Numerous candidate genes have been studied for their role in risk for the disorder.[46]

Ongoing biological studies suggest fundamental disturbances in serotonergic function in individuals with BN.[80,84] The ultimate understanding of the etiology of BN and of other disturbances that contribute to the development of inappropriate responses to satiety clues[85] will most likely include main effects of both biological and environmental factors as well as their interactions and correlations.

Course of Illness

Although BN is not typically associated with the serious physical complications normally associated with AN, patients commonly report physical symptoms such as fatigue, lethargy, bloating, and gastrointestinal problems. Individuals with BN who engage in frequent vomiting may experience electrolyte abnormalities, metabolic alkalosis, erosion of dental enamel, swelling of the parotid glands, and scars and calluses on the backs of their hands.[86] Those who frequently misuse laxatives can have edema, fluid loss and subsequent dehydration, electrolyte abnormalities, metabolic acidosis, and potentially permanent loss of normal bowel function.[86] Chapter 6 reviews eating-related, psychological, and biomarker-measured outcomes of BN in detail.

Treatment

In the United States, most treatment for BN is conducted on an outpatient basis. Given the frequency of medical[87] and nutritional complications, a comprehensive medical evaluation is the typical first step in treatment. Thereafter, psychotherapy, delivered either individually or in group format, is usually the cornerstone of BN interventions. Common approaches include cognitive-behavioral therapy and interpersonal psychotherapy. In cases in which the individual is experiencing medical complications of BN, is pregnant, or is unable to bring an entrenched binge-purge cycle under control on an outpatient basis, partial hospitalization or inpatient treatment is often warranted.

In 1996, the Food and Drug Administration (FDA) approved fluoxetine for the treatment of BN. Currently, this is the only FDA-approved medication for the treatment of any eating disorder.

Eating Disorders Not Otherwise Specified (Binge Eating Disorder)

Clinical Characteristics

Eating disorders not otherwise specified (EDNOS) is a diagnostic category that captures those individuals with eating disorders who do not meet criteria for AN or BN. The DSM IV lists six different examples of presentations of EDNOS:

1. all features of AN except amenorrhea;
2. all features of AN except remaining in a normal weight range;
3. all criteria for BN except frequency of binge eating or purging or duration of 3 months;
4. regular inappropriate compensatory behavior after eating small amounts of food;
5. chewing and spitting out food; and
6. binge eating disorder (BED).

Clinical reports suggest that individuals with EDNOS constitute the majority of individuals seeking professional help for an eating disorder.[88,89] This suggests that the nomenclature for eating disorders is imperfect. Moreover, our attempts to address the key questions of this evidence report for the global category of EDNOS indicated a paucity of investigations on the nature of the highly heterogeneous category of EDNOS and on the treatment and outcome of specific presentations of EDNOS. We redirected the task to focus on BED, the one category of EDNOS that has a corpus of research.

Diagnostic Criteria

The symptom of binge eating was first recognized in a subset of obese individuals by Stunkard in 1959.[90] BED has had a slow and controversial evolution in the psychiatric nosology for eating disorders.[91-94] DSM IV currently includes BED as a disorder requiring further study.

The DSM IV criteria appear in Table 3. Individuals with BED engage in regular binge eating behavior. A binge eating episode is determined in the same manner as in BN; it requires consumption of an unusually large amount of food and a sense of being out of control. The frequency criterion of twice per week is the same as in BN, although this criterion is not well supported by the literature.[95,96] Unlike BN, individuals with BED do not regularly engage in compensatory behaviors. Several other criteria in the provisional BED diagnosis require further empirical support.

Table 3. Diagnostic criteria: binge eating disorder

Diagnostic Criteria	
DSM IV Criteria for Binge Eating Disorder (307.50)	A. Recurrent episodes of binge eating. An episode of binge eating is characterized by both of the following: (1) Eating, in a discrete period of time (e.g., within any 2-hour period), an amount of food that is definitely larger than most people would eat in a similar period of time under similar circumstances (2) The sense of lack of control over eating during the episode (e.g., a feeling that one cannot stop eating or control what or how much one is eating) B. Binge-eating episodes are associated with three (or more) of the following: (1) eating much more rapidly than normal (2) eating until feeling uncomfortably full (3) eating large amounts of food when not feeling physically hungry (4) eating along because of being embarrassed by how much one is eating (5) feeling disgusted with oneself, depressed, or very guilty after overeating C. Marked distress regarding binge eating is present D. The binge eating occurs, on average, at least 2 days a week for 6 months Note: The method of determining frequency differs from that used for bulimia nervosa; future research should address whether the preferred method of setting a frequency threshold is counting the number of days on which binges occur or counting the number of episodes of binge eating E. The binge eating is not associated with the regular use of inappropriate compensatory behavior (e.g., purging, fasting, excessive exercise, etc.) and does not occur exclusively during the course of anorexia nervosa or bulimia nervosa

DSM, Diagnostic and Statistical Manual.

Epidemiology

Population-based studies suggest that between 0.7 percent and 3 percent of individuals in community samples meet criteria for BED.[92,97-99] Community studies of obese individuals have found a prevalence of BED between 5 percent and 8 percent.[100,101] Population-based studies of

BED and the component behavior of binge eating report a relatively equal gender distribution,[92,99] few differences in prevalence across races or ethnic groups,[102] and possibly increased risk associated with lower socioeconomic status.[103,104] In a population-based study of female twins, 37 percent of obese women (BMI ≥ 30) endorsed the symptom of binge eating,[105] representing 2.7 percent of the female population studied.

Etiology

In a community-based case-control study, Fairburn et al.[106] found significant differences in exposure to risk factors between women with BED and healthy controls, but surprisingly few differences between women with BED and BN. In comparison to healthy controls, women with BED reported greater adverse childhood experiences, parental depression, personal vulnerability to depression, and exposure to negative comments about weight, shape, and eating.

BED has been shown to aggregate in families.[107] Although heritability estimates for frank BED are not yet available, the heritability of binge eating in the absence of compensatory behaviors has been estimated to be 41 percent.[108] In addition, binge eating has been explored as a potential intermediate behavioral phenotype in understanding the genetics of obesity. It has also been preliminarily identified in some studies as an important phenotypic characteristic of individuals with a mutation in the melanocortin 4 receptor (*MC4R*), a candidate gene that influences eating behavior,[109] although this finding has not been replicated.[110]

Course of Illness

Given that BED has only recently entered the psychiatric nomenclature, we have minimal population-based data on morbidity and mortality. The presence of binge eating or BED in obese individuals carries substantial risk. Obese individuals with binge eating or BED in clinical and community studies report earlier onsets of obesity and dieting,[92,111,112] greater weight fluctuations,[112] more cognitive features of disordered eating,[113] lower self-esteem and self-efficacy,[114] and higher scores on depression indices.[114-117] Chapter 6 reviews eating-related, psychological, and biomarker-measured outcomes of BED in detail.

Treatment

In the United States, treatment for BED is typically conducted on an outpatient basis. Psychological and dietary interventions aim to reduce binge eating and control weight.[118] Common psychotherapeutic approaches include cognitive-behavioral and interpersonal psychotherapy; nutritional approaches include very low calorie diets and behavioral self-management strategies.[118] Pharmacotherapy targeting both the core symptoms of binge eating and weight loss are also available as off-label interventions.[119]

Production of This Evidence Report

Organization

Given that eating disorders are an important public health problem, the Agency for Healthcare Research and Quality (AHRQ), the National Institutes of Health's Office of Research on Women's Health, together with the Health Resources and Services Administration (HRSA), and in consultation with National Institute of Mental Health (NIMH), commissioned an evidence report through its Evidence Based Practice Program and assigned it to the RTI International-University of North Carolina Evidence-Based Practice Center (RTI-UNC EPC). The issue is also of particular concern to the American Psychiatric Association and the Laureate Psychiatric Clinic and Hospital, which nominated the topic.

Chapter 2 describes our methodological approach, including the development of key questions and their analytic framework, our search strategies, and inclusion/exclusion criteria. In Chapters 3 through 5, we separately present the results of our literature search and synthesis on the treatment of each disease (respectively, AN, BN, and BED). Chapter 6 documents our findings about outcomes associated with each disease. Chapter 7 further discusses our findings, grades the strength of the bodies of literature, highlights methodological shortcomings of the extant research, and offers recommendations for future research. Appendixes (available electronically at http://www.ahrq.gov) provide a detailed description of our search strings (Appendix A[*]), our quality rating forms (Appendix B), detailed evidence tables (Appendix C), list of excluded studies (Appendix D), and acknowledgments including our Technical Expert Panel and peer reviewers (Appendix E).

Technical Expert Panel

We identified experts in the field of eating disorders to provide assistance throughout the project. The Technical Expert Panel (TEP) (see Appendix E) contributes to AHRQ's broader goals of (1) creating and maintaining science partnerships as well as public-private partnerships and (2) meeting the needs of an array of potential customers and users of this product. The TEP served as both a resource and sounding board during the project. Our TEP comprised 10 individuals: three psychiatrists and two psychologists with eating disorder expertise; two nurses; one pediatric/adolescent medicine physician; one nutritionist; and one patient advocate.

To ensure accountability and scientifically relevant work, the TEP was called upon to provide guidance at all stages of the project. TEP members participated in conference calls and e-mail exchanges to

- refine the analytic framework and key questions at the beginning of the project;
- refine the scope of the project; and
- discuss inclusion and exclusion criteria.

Because of their extensive knowledge of the literature on eating disorders, including numerous articles authored by TEP members, and their active involvement in professional organizations and as practitioners in the field, we also asked TEP members to participate in external peer review of the draft report.

Uses of This Report

We anticipate this report will be of value to members of the various professional organizations who treat eating disorders. These include the Academy for Eating Disorders, American Academy of Pediatrics, American Academy of Family Practice, American College of Obstetricians and Gynecologists, American Dietetics Association, American Psychiatric Association, American Psychological Association, International Association of Eating Disorders Professionals, National Association of Social Workers, and Society for Adolescent Medicine.

---

[*] Appendixes cited in this report are provided electronically at
http://www.ahrq.gov/downloads/pub/evidence/pdf/eatingdisorders/eatdis.pdf.

More generally, the report will assist these organizations in their mission to inform and educate practitioners. From this review, the National Institutes of Health can identify serious gaps in the research on eating disorders to guide funding policy. It can inform practitioners on the current evidence about outcomes associated with having these eating disorders and treating patients with them. Researchers will benefit from the concise analysis of the current status of the field, which will enable them to design future studies to address deficiencies in the field. Health educators can use this report to improve health communication. Finally, policymakers can use this report to allocate resources toward future research and initiatives that are likely to be successful.

Chapter 2. Methods

In this chapter, we document the procedures that the RTI International – University of North Carolina at Chapel Hill Evidence-based Practice Center (RTI-UNC EPC) used to develop this comprehensive evidence report on the management and outcomes related to eating disorders. To provide a framework for the review, we first present the key questions and their underlying analytic framework. We then describe our strategy for identifying articles relevant to our key questions, our inclusion/exclusion criteria, and the process we used to abstract relevant information from eligible articles and generate our evidence tables. We also discuss our criteria for grading the quality of individual articles and the strength of the evidence as a whole. Last, we explain the peer review process.

Key Questions and Analytic Framework

This report spans key questions (KQs) regarding both treatment and outcomes of three eating disorders: anorexia nervosa (AN), bulimia nervosa (BN), and eating disorders not otherwise specified (EDNOS), which we refined to focus exclusively on binge eating disorder (BED) because of the lack of availability of data on other EDNOS conditions. We examine issues concerning treatment efficacy and disease outcomes separately for each disorder. The American Psychiatric Association and Laureate Psychiatric Clinic and Hospital initially offered these questions, and we put them into final form with input from our Technical Expert Panel (TEP).

Key Questions

- 1. What is the evidence for the efficacy of treatments or combination of treatments for each of the following eating disorders: AN, BN, and BED?
- 2. What is the evidence of harms associated with the treatment or combination of treatments for each of the following eating disorders: AN, BN, and BED?
- 3. What factors are associated with the efficacy of treatment among patients with the following eating disorders: AN, BN, and BED?
- 4. Does the efficacy of treatment for AN, BN, and BED differ by sex, gender, age, race, ethnicity, or cultural group?
- 5. What factors are associated with outcomes among individuals with the following eating disorders: AN, BN, and BED?
- 6. Do outcomes for AN, BN, and BED differ by sex, gender, age, race, ethnicity, or cultural group?

In the analytic framework for these questions (Figure 1), we depict the partially overlapping syndromes of AN, BN and BED, the two types of studies included in this review (treatment and outcome analyses), and factors that influence both treatment response and disorder outcome. We do not include in our figure influencing factors, such as physical and sexual abuse, that are not discussed in the literature meeting our inclusion criteria.

Also depicted on the framework are the six KQs discussed in this report. KQ 1 addresses the efficacy of available treatments for the three disorders; we categorize outcomes as eating-related

Figure 1. Analytic framework

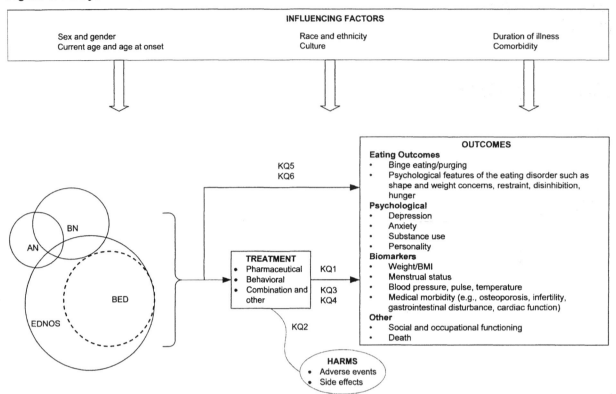

outcomes that deal with the core behavioral and psychological pathology of the disorders, psychiatric or psychological outcomes that focus on the presence of comorbid depression and anxiety, and biomarker outcomes that reflect weight, body mass index (BMI), and other biological indices of the disorders. Treatment may include relapse, diagnostic crossover, and symptomatic change. KQ 2 explores the harms associated with both medication and psychological treatments for these disorders. KQs 3 and 4 highlight the roles of illness-related factors (e.g., comorbid depression, subtype of the eating disorders, early onset of illness) and illness-independent factors (e.g., sex, gender, race or ethnicity, age) in influencing the outcomes of treating these conditions.

KQ 5 addresses short- and long-term outcomes of the disorders. We apply information from observational, cohort, and case series investigations and focus on eating-related, psychiatric or psychological, and biological indices. Finally, KQ 6 highlights whether these outcomes differ by sex, gender, age, race or ethnicity, or cultural groups.

Literature Review Methods

Inclusion and Exclusion Criteria

After discussions with our TEP, we generated a list of article inclusion and exclusion criteria (Table 4) for these KQs. We limited our review to human studies, including participants ages 10 years and older. Although interest is growing in developing appropriate nomenclature and interventions for young children with eating disorders,[120] we judged this literature to be beyond the scope of this review. We considered studies published in all languages from 1980 to

September 2005. We included studies conducted with participants of both sexes, in all nations. The study population must be primarily diagnosed with AN, BN or BED.

Table 4. Eating disorders literature searches: inclusion and exclusion criteria

Category	Criteria
Study population	Humans All races, ethnicities, and cultural groups 10 years of age or older.
Study settings and geography	All nations
Time period	Published from 1980 to the present
Publication criteria	All languages Articles in print Articles in the "gray literature," published in nonpeer-reviewed journals, or unobtainable during the review period were excluded.
Admissible evidence (study design and other criteria)	Original research studies that provide sufficient detail regarding methods and results to enable use and adjustment of the data and results. Anorexia nervosa must be diagnosed according to DSM III, DSM III-R, DSM IV, ICD-10, Feighner, or Russell criteria. Bulimia nervosa must be diagnosed according to DSM III-R, DSM IV, or ICD-10 criteria. Eating disorders not otherwise specified (binge eating disorder) must be diagnosed according to DSM IV criteria. Relevant outcomes: eating related, psychiatric or psychological, and biomarker measures; must be able to be abstracted from data presented in the papers. Eligible study designs include: **Randomized controlled trials (RCTs):** Double-blinded, single-blinded, and cross-over designs (data from prior to the first cross-over). Anorexia nervosa studies: initiated with 10 or more participants and followed for any length of time. Eating disorders not otherwise specified (binge eating disorder) studies: initiated with 10 or more participants and followed for any length of time. Bulimia nervosa studies: initiated with 30 or more patients and followed for a minimum of 3 months. **Outcomes studies:** Observational studies including prospective and retrospective cohort studies and case series studies, with and without comparison populations. Disease population must be followed for a minimum of 1 year. Disease population must include 50 or more participants at the time of the analysis.

We excluded data that combined diseases because such mixed information would preclude us from separately examining evidence on any one of the three conditions. We also excluded editorials, letters, and commentaries; articles that did not report outcomes related to our key questions; and studies that did not provide sufficient information to be abstracted. Studies were required to report on at least one of our outcomes categories of interest: eating, psychiatric and psychological, or biomarker measures.

We defined individuals as having one of the three disorders of interest according to specific diagnostic criteria. We examined the impact of treatment through a review of the RCT efficacy of treatment literature.

To address a TEP concern that the size of the available AN and BED literature was too limited to permit us to constrain this review based on sample size or followup duration, we included very small AN and BED RCT treatment studies in our review (10 or more participants) and did not require specified followup durations for a study to be included. The BN literature, however, is much more voluminous, which allowed us to limit the treatment studies to larger ones (i.e., those with 30 or more participants).

To help ensure that we were not measuring short-term fluctuations in disease symptoms, we required BN efficacy of treatment studies to follow patients for a minimum of 3 months. The decision to place more stringent requirements on the BN literature was made in consultation with our TEP. Because of financial and time considerations, we used a recently completed EPC report entitled *Drug Class Review on Second Generation Antidepressants*[121] as a starting point for our discussion of harms or side effects related to *receiving treatment* for AN, BN, and BED; we then supplemented this information with harms reported in the RCT studies meeting our inclusion criteria.

We examined outcomes related to having one of the three eating disorders through a review of observational studies; outcomes included eating, psychiatric or psychological, and biomarker variables and death. Although many participants followed in these studies have received treatment, the outcomes of interest relate not to efficacy of treatments but rather to disease levels and other problems that persist over time. To avoid reporting short-term fluctuations among the disease populations and to have sufficient sample sizes to observe changes over time, we limited our review to studies of 50 or more individuals, followed for a minimum of 1 year, with or without comparison groups. Our TEP concurred with this plan.

For both the RCT and outcome literatures, we were unable to perform pooled meta-analyses. Given the absence of consensus definitions of remission, recovery, and relapse for eating disorders, as well as the overabundance of outcome measures, we judged meta-analysis to be both inadvisable and infeasible.

Literature Search and Retrieval Process

Databases and search terms. To identify the relevant literature for our review, we conducted systematic searches based on search terms, reviewed included studies by our TEP, and hand searched reference lists. We searched standard electronic databases such as MEDLINE®, the Cumulative Index to Nursing and Applied Health (CINAHL), PsycINFO, the Educational Resources Information Center (ERIC), the National AGRICultural OnLine Access (AGRICOLA), and Cochrane Collaboration libraries.

Based on inclusion/exclusion criteria specified above, we generated a list of Medical Subject Heading (MeSH) search terms, supplemented by key word searches of MEDLINE®. Comparable terms were used to search other databases. MeSH terms included anorexia, anorexia nervosa, and bulimia. Text terms included binge eating disorder. We limited our searches by type of study, including RCT, single-blind method, double-blind method, random allocation, longitudinal studies, and observational studies. For interventions, we used therapeutics or cognitive therapy or family therapy or drug therapy or therapy, computer-assisted. For outcomes of disease, we used outcome assessment (health care), treatment outcome, outcome and process assessment (health care), and recurrence. Finally, we asked our external peer reviewers for titles of articles that we may have missed.

Figure 2 presents the yield and results from our searches. We conducted our initial search in late 2004 and updated it in August 2005 (treatment studies) and September 2005 (outcome studies). Beginning with a yield of 2,188 titles and abstracts, we reviewed and further narrowed this pool to 478 articles.

Figure 2. Eating disorders article disposition

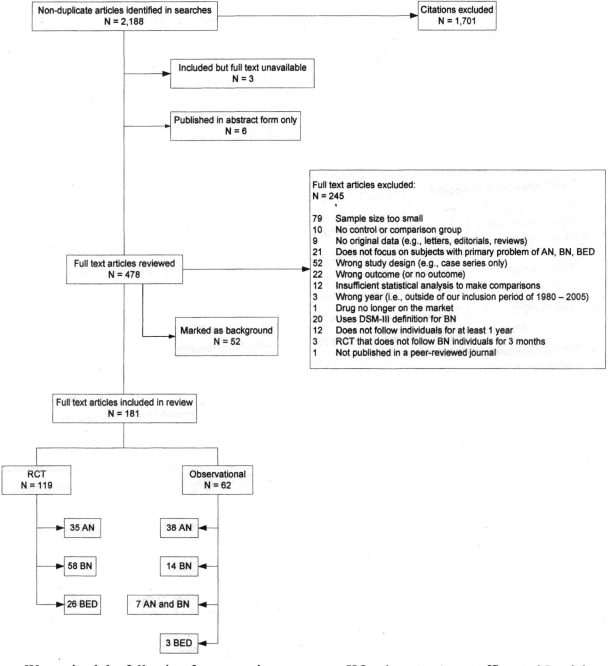

We retained the following for our review to answer KQs about treatment efficacy: 35 articles on AN, 58 articles on BN, and 26 articles on BED. To answer KQs about disease outcomes, we retained 38 articles on AN, 14 articles on BN, 7 articles on both AN and BN, and 3 articles on BED.

Article selection process. Once we had identified articles through the electronic database search, review articles, and bibliographies, we examined titles and abstracts to determine whether the studies met our inclusion criteria. One reviewer initially evaluated abstracts for inclusion or exclusion. If one reviewer concluded that the article should be included, it was retained. Abstracts initially excluded from the study by one reviewer received a second review by senior project staff—Nancy Berkman, PhD, MLIR (Project Director), Cynthia Bulik, PhD (Scientific Director), or Gerald Gartlehner, MD, MPH (UNC Project Manager).

In all, 478 articles appeared to meet our inclusion criteria through abstract review, so we obtained the full articles. For the full article review, one senior reviewer read each article and determined if it met our eligibility criteria. Those articles that the reviewer determined did not meet our criteria were re-reviewed by a second senior reviewer to ensure agreement that the article should be excluded. We assigned each of these articles one or more reasons for exclusion.

Literature Synthesis

Development of Evidence Tables and Data Abstraction Process

The senior staff members for this systematic review jointly developed the evidence tables. We created two designs for the evidence tables, one for KQs 1 to 4 (treatment studies) and one for KQs 5 and 6 (outcome studies). They are intended to provide sufficient information for readers to understand the study and determine its quality; we emphasized presenting information essential to answering the main questions. The formats of the two sets of evidence tables were based on successful designs used for prior systematic reviews.

Columns in the evidence tables for treatment studies report baseline and outcome measures for eating-related, psychological or psychiatric, and biomarker variables. For each outcome measured, the tables present data in a consistent format. Given the large number of outcomes that these studies typically report, our evidence table entries are relatively long. In contrast, the outcome studies evidence tables are shorter. However, because of the appreciable variety of study approaches and outcomes reported in this literature the presentation of outcome data is, by necessity, less consistent than that for the treatment studies.

For this work, the RTI-UNC EPC team decided to abstract data from included articles directly into evidence tables; this system has worked effectively in many of our past reviews. Because we bypassed the use of data abstraction forms, we had significant efficiencies in production.

We trained data abstractors intensively, thoroughly familiarizing them with table designs, required information and formats, and examples of abstracted articles. As the work progressed, we shared various reporting requirements with abstractors to ensure that information appeared in a consistent and easily understandable manner.

For both the treatment and the outcomes literatures, the first reviewer (UNC faculty, postdoctoral psychology fellow, or psychology graduate student) initially entered data from the article into the evidence table. The second reviewer (Drs. Berkman, Bulik, Brownley, Carey, or Gartlehner) read the article and edited the initial table entry for accuracy, completeness, and consistency. All disagreements concerning the information reported in the evidence tables were reconciled by the two abstractors.

The final evidence tables are presented in their entirety in Appendix C.[*] Separate tables are included for treatment studies by disease and type of treatment intervention:

- AN: Evidence Table 1, medication trials; Evidence Table 2, medication plus behavioral intervention trials; Evidence Table 3, behavioral intervention trials (adults); and Evidence Table 4, behavioral intervention trials (adolescents ages 10 and older);
- BN: Evidence Table 5, medication trials; Evidence Table 6, medication plus behavioral intervention trials; Evidence Table 7, behavior intervention with no medications trials; Evidence Table 8, self-help interventions trials; and Evidence Table 9, other interventions trials;
- BED: Evidence Table 10, medication trials; Evidence Table 11, medication plus behavioral interventions trials; Evidence Table 12, behavioral intervention with no medications trials; Evidence Table 13, self-help intervention trials; and Evidence Table 14, other interventions trials.

Appendix C also presents three evidence tables for outcome studies organized only by disease:

- AN outcome studies, Evidence Table 15;
- BN outcome studies, Evidence Table 16; and
- BED outcome studies, Evidence Table 17.

Within each evidence table, entries are listed alphabetically by the last name of the first author. Abbreviations and acronyms used in the tables appear in a glossary at the beginning of the appendix.

Finally, as noted earlier, the number of assessment instruments that investigators used for both diagnosis and outcome measurement in the studies reviewed here was extremely large. To help readers identify these, we created Table 5 (found at the end of this chapter) to briefly identify all measures, their acronyms or abbreviations, and their subscales, with a citation to a definitive source for the instrument.

Quality and Strength of Evidence Evaluation

Rating the quality of individual articles. For this systematic review, we developed our approach to assessing the quality of individual articles using domains and elements recommended in the evidence report by West and colleagues, *Systems to Rate the Strength of Scientific Evidence*.[122] We developed two quality-rating forms, one for the treatment literature and the other for the outcomes literature. Quality rating forms did not differ by disease. We tested several drafts of these forms, revising them as needed to ensure that they efficiently captured the desired information. The final grading forms can be found in Appendix B.

We assessed the treatment literature through 25 items in 11 categories: (1) research aim/study question, (2) study population, (3) randomization, (4) blinding, (5) interventions, (6) outcomes, (7) statistical analysis, (8) results, (9) discussion, (10) external validity, and (11) funding/sponsorship. We did not exclude any studies with so-called fatal flaws, such as the approach to randomization. Rather, we reduced the study's overall score if a category was flawed

---

[*] Appendixes cited in this report are provided electronically at
http://www.ahrq.gov/downloads/pub/evidence/pdf/eatingdisorders/eatdis.pdf.

or inadequate. Because patients and those administering interventions in the psychological treatment studies could not be blinded, we did not evaluate these items when studies included these interventions. However, we always evaluated whether the outcome assessor was blinded. Studies that were reported in more than one article were given the same quality grade.

We weighted each item equally and calculated a score out of 100 percent. We then collapsed those scores into three categories: poor, 0 percent to 59 percent; fair, 60 percent to 74 percent; and good, 75 percent or better.

For the outcomes literature, we used 17 items in 8 categories: (1) research aim/study question, (2) study population, (3) eating disorder diagnosis method, (4) study design, (5) statistical analysis, (6) results/outcome measurement, (7) external validity, and (8) discussion. As with the RCTs, we weighted each item equally. Rather than calculating a score out of 100 percent, however, we converted ratings for each item into numeric values of 0, 1, or 2, in which 0 = poor, 1 = fair, and 2 = good. Studies without comparison groups were not evaluated by items addressing this aspect of design. However, studies that included comparison groups were scored as "good" on one item, whereas those without were scored as "poor" on that item. We calculated the mean score for all graded items and we concluded that, overall, an article should be graded as poor with a rating < 1, fair with a rating ≥ 1 and < 1.5, and good with a rating of ≥ 1.5.

Each quality grade was the composite (averaged) rating of two independent evaluators. The only items reconciled between the evaluators were those in which one rater provided a score for the item and the other said the item was not applicable. In assessing quality of the treatment studies, we asked the two evaluators to discuss their results if the difference in their total scores was 20 points or greater, but we did not require them to come to agreement.

Rating the strength of the available evidence. We rated the strength of the evidence base for both interventions and disease outcomes separately for the three diseases, using a single scheme for all bodies of evidence. Starting with the West et al. report that compared various schemes for grading bodies of evidence,[122] we based our evaluation on criteria developed by Greer et al.,[123] which we deemed most applicable to the study designs in this review. It includes three domains: quality of the research, quantity of studies (including number of studies and adequacy of the sample size), and consistency of findings.

We graded the body of literature applicable to each of the six KQs separately. For the treatment literature, we further divided studies by whether the intervention was pharmaceutical, behavioral, or a combination. Three senior staff defined by consensus four strength-of-evidence categories, as follows:

I.   Strong evidence base. The evidence is from studies of strong design; results are both clinically important and consistent with minor exceptions at most; results are free from serious doubts about generalizability, bias, or flaws in research design. Studies with negative results have sufficiently large samples to have adequate statistical power.

II.   Moderate evidence base. The evidence is from studies of strong design, but some uncertainty remains because of inconsistencies or concern about generalizability, bias, research design flaws, or adequate sample size. Alternatively, the evidence is consistent but derives from studies of weaker design.

III. Weak evidence base. The evidence is from a limited number of studies of weaker design. Studies with strong design either have not been done or are inconclusive.

IV.   No evidence base. No published literature.

Peer Review Process

Among the more important activities involved in producing a credible evidence report is conducting an unbiased and broadly based review of the draft report. External reviewers for this report included clinicians, representatives of professional societies and advocacy groups, and potential users of the report, including TEP members (see Appendix D[†]). We charged peer reviewers with commenting on the content, structure, and format of the evidence report and asked them to complete a peer review checklist. We revised the report, as appropriate, based on their comments.

[†] Appendixes cited in this report are provided electronically at
http://www.ahrq.gov/downloads/pub/evidence/pdf/eatingdisorders/eatdis.pdf.

Table 5. Diagnostic and outcome measures used in randomized controlled trials and outcome studies

Acronym and Full Name of Test	Description of Test and Subscales
ABOS: Anorectic Behaviour Scale for Inpatient Observation[124]	Proxy-report (relatives) questionnaire to obtain information about patient's behaviors and attitudes; 3 factors: eating behaviors, concerns with weight and food, denial of proteins; bulimic-like behaviors; hyperactivity.
ABS: Anorectic Behavior Scale[125]	Administrator-completed questionnaire about patient's behavior while in hospital; 8 items on resistance to eating, 8 items on methods of disposing of food, 6 items on overactivity.
ANSS: Anorexia Nervosa Symptom Score[126]	Clinical rating scale with psychological, social, and physical severity scores and subscales.
BAT: Body Attitudes Test[127,128]	Self-report questionnaire to measure subjective body experience and attitude towards one's body; 3 factors: negative attitudes about body size, lack of familiarity with one's own body, body dissatisfaction.
BDI: Beck Depression Inventory[129]	One of the most widely used self-report measures for depression. It is a 21-item test presented in multiple choice format that measures the presence and degree of depression in adolescents and adults.
BEDCI: Binge Eating Disorder Clinical Interview[130]	Structured clinical interview to establish the diagnosis of BED and both purging and nonpurging types of BN.
BES: Binge Eating Scale[131]	Self-report measure of binge eating severity as measured by loss of control over eating behavior; 8 items on behavioral manifestations, 8 items on feelings and cognitions.
BIAQ: Body Image Avoidance Questionnaire[132]	Self-report measure to assess avoidance of situations that provoke concern about physical appearance (including wearing tight fitting clothing, social outings, physical intimacy); 4 subscales: Eating Restraint, Clothing, Grooming/Weighing, Social Activities
BITE: Bulimic Investigation Test Edinburgh[133]	Brief self-report questionnaire with 2 subscales designed to assess the symptoms and severity of binge eating episodes.
BSI: Brief Symptom Inventory[134]	Brief self-report instrument to assess patients at intake for psychiatric problems; 9 Primary Symptom Dimensions: Somatization, Obsessive-Compulsive, Interpersonal Sensitivity, Depression, Anxiety, Hostility, Phobic Anxiety, Paranoid Ideation, Psychoticism; 3 Global Indices: Global Severity Index, Positive Symptom Distress Index, Positive Symptom Total.
BSQ: Body Shape Questionnaire[135]	Self-report inventory to measure worries about weight and body shape.
BSQ-short version: Body Shape Questionnaire – Short Version[136]	Self-report inventory to measure worries about weight and body shape.
BSS: Body Satisfaction Scale[137]	Self-report instrument to assess body image satisfaction; 3 subscales: general, body, head.
Bulimic Thoughts Questionnaire[138]	Self-report instrument of cognitive patterns and distortions associated with bulimic behavior.
CBCL: Child Behavior Checklist[139]	Parent-report standardized assessment of behavioral problems and social competencies of children ages 4 to 18; 3 scores: total, internalizing behaviors (fearful, shy, anxious, inhibited), externalizing behaviors (aggressive, antisocial, under controlled).
CCEI: Crown-Crisp Experimental Index[140]	Scale to measure neurotic symptomatology; 6 subscales: free-floating anxiety, phobic anxiety, obsessionality, somatic concomitants of anxiety, depression, hysterical personality.
CDI: Children's Depression Inventory[141]	Brief self-report test to measure cognitive, affective, and behavioral signs of depression in persons 6 to 17 years of age; 5 factors: negative mood, interpersonal problems, ineffectiveness, anhedonia, negative self-esteem.

Table 5. Diagnostic and outcome measures used in randomized controlled trials and outcome studies (continued)

Acronym and Full Name of Test	Description of Test and Subscales
CDRS: Contour Drawing Rating Scale[142]	Instrument to assess body size perception and dissatisfaction; 9 male and 9 female contour drawings shown to subjects who are asked to indicate which most closely resembles their current size and their ideal figure; the discrepancy is a measure of body dissatisfaction in 3 scores: real body, ideal body, body satisfaction index.
CGI or GIS: Clinical Global Impression[143]	Clinician-rated scale to assess treatment response in psychiatric patients; 3 subscales: severity of illness (CGI-S), global improvement (CSI-G), efficacy index (CGI-EI).
DICA-R: Diagnostic Interview for Children and Adolescents – Revised[144]	Semistructured clinical interview to determine Axis I psychiatric diagnoses in children and adolescents.
DIET: Dieter's Inventory of Eating Temptations[145]	Self-report inventory to assess behavioral competence in 6 weight control situations: overeating, negative emotions, exercise, resisting temptation, positive social, food choice.
DSED: Diagnostic Survey for Eating Disorders[146]	Self-report questionnaire to quantify frequency of disturbed behavior.
EAT: Eating Attitudes Test[147]	Standardized self-report measure of symptoms and concern characteristics of eating disorders; 2 versions: EAT-26, EAT-40.
EDE: Eating Disorder Examination[148]	Semistructured interview to measure specific psychopathology of anorexia nervosa and bulimia nervosa; 4 subscales: dietary restraint, eating concern, weight concern, shape concern.
EDE-Q4: Eating Disorders Evaluation Questionnaire – Version 4[149]	Self-report assessment of thoughts and behaviors commonly found in eating disorders; 4 subscales: dietary restraint, eating concern, weight concern, shape concern.
EDI-1: Eating Disorder Inventory-1[149]	Self-report questionnaire to measure psychiatric and behavioral traits commonly associated with eating disorders; 8 scales: drive for thinness, bulimia, body dissatisfaction, ineffectiveness, perfectionism, interpersonal distrust, interoceptive awareness, maturity fears.
EDI-2: Eating Disorder Inventory- 2[150]	Standardized self-report measure of psychiatric symptoms commonly associated with anorexia nervosa, bulimia nervosa, or other eating disorders; 8 subscales as for EDI-1, plus asceticism, impulse regulation, and social insecurity.
FACES III: Family Adaptability and Cohesion Evaluation Scales[151]	Instrument to assess family adaptation and cohesion. Family cohesion assesses degree of separation or connection of family members to the family; 4 levels of family cohesion range from extreme low cohesion to extreme high cohesion: disengaged, separated, connected, enmeshed; 4 levels of adaptability: rigid, structured, flexible, chaotic.
FAM III: Family Assessment Measure[152]	Self-report measure that assesses the strengths and weaknesses of functioning within a family; can be completed by pre-adolescents, adolescents, and adult family members (ages 10 years to adult); contains 7 subscales: Task Accomplishment, Role Performance, Communication, Affective Expression, Involvement, Control, Values and Norms.
FES: Family Environment Scale[153]	Instrument to assess actual, preferred, and expected social environment of all types of families; 10 subscales: cohesion, expressiveness, conflict, independence, achievement, intellectual-cultural, active-recreation, moral-religious, organization, control.
FMPS: Frost Multidimensional Perfectionism Scale[154]	Self-report measure of perfectionism; original measure had 6 subscales (Concern Over Mistakes, Personal Standards, Parental Expectations, Parental Criticism, Doubts About Actions, Organization).
FNE: Fear of Negative Evaluation[155,156]	Scale to measure social anxiety about receiving negative evaluations from others; 2 subscales: Negative Expectations, Negative Public Evaluation.
Brief-FNE: Brief Fear of Negative Evaluation[157]	Brief version of the original FNE.

Table 5. Diagnostic and outcome measures used in randomized controlled trials and outcome studies (continued)

Acronym and Full Name of Test	Description of Test and Subscales
FRS: Figure Rating Scale[158]	Silhouette drawings of male and female adult body figures ranging from very thin to very large used as measure of personal body perception; 3 subscales: Real Body, Ideal Body, Body Satisfaction Index.
GAAS: Goldberg Anorectic Attitude Scale[159]	Scale to measure short-term changes in anorectic cognitions across treatment including measures of hyperactivity, access, self-care, selective appetite, and denial of illness.
GAF: Global Assessment of Functioning[16]	Clinician-derived instrument to measure the highest level of social and occupational functioning in the previous week and year; sometimes broken down into the GAF-F function score (not including symptoms) and the GAF-S symptom score (not including function).
GIS: Global Improvement Scale[143]	See CGI (Clinical Global Improvement Scale).
HAM-A: Hamilton Anxiety Rating Scale[160]	Semistructured interview to assess severity of anxiety symptomatology.
HAM-D or HDRS: Hamilton Depression Rating Scale[161]	Semistructured interview to assess an array of behavioral, affective, and vegetative symptoms of depression.
HGSHS: Harvard Group Scale of Hypnotic Susceptibility, Form A[162]	Measure of susceptibility to a wide range of hypnotic experiences, designed for assessing groups of subjects.
HRQ: Helping Relationship Questionnaire[163]	Patient-rated instrument to measure therapeutic alliance.
HSCL: Hopkins Symptom Checklist[134]	Self-report screening instrument to identify common psychiatric symptoms; 9 subscales: somatization, obsessive–compulsive symptoms, interpersonal sensitivity, depression, anxiety, anger or hostility, phobic anxiety, paranoid ideation, psychotic symptoms.
IBC: Interactive Behavior Code[164]	A global interferential measure of communication, problem solving, and conflict, with 22 coded items rated by independent observers; summary scores are computed for negative and positive communication.
IIP: Inventory of Interpersonal Problems[165]	Instrument to measure interpersonal problems and level of distress arising from interpersonal sources.
LCB: Locus of Control of Behavior[166]	Instrument to measure the extent to which individuals believe they are responsible for personal problem behavior.
LIFE: Longitudinal Interval Continuation Evaluation[167]	Semistructured interview and rating system to assess longitudinal course of psychiatric disorders in several areas: psychopathology, nonpsychiatric mental illness, treatment, psychosocial functioning, overall severity, narrative account.
MCMI: Millon Clinical Multiaxial Inventory[168]	Lengthy test to diagnose 14 personality disorders and 10 clinical syndromes; scales: 14 Personality Pattern Scales, 10 Clinical Syndrome Scales, 3 Modifying Indices, 1 Validity Index.
MMPI: Minnesota Multiphasic Personality Inventory[169]	Test of adult psychopathology; 8 Validity Scales, 5 Superlative Self-Presentation Subscales, 10 Clinical Scales, 9 Restructured Clinical (RC) Scales, 15 Content Scales, 27 Content Component Scales, 20 Supplementary Scales, 31 Clinical Subscales (Harris-Lingoes and Social Introversion Subscales), and various special or setting-specific indices.
MOCI: Maudsley Obsessive Compulsive Index[170]	Self-report questionnaire to measure the presence of obsessional-compulsive behaviors; scores: total obsessional symptoms; checking; washing; doubting/conscientious; slowness/repetition.
MPS: Multidimensional Perfectionism Scale[154]	Self-report instrument to assess perfectionism; 6 subscales: concern over mistakes, personal standards, parental expectations, parental criticism, doubts about action, organization.

Table 5. Diagnostic and outcome measures used in randomized controlled trials and outcome studies (continued)

Acronym and Full Name of Test	Description of Test and Subscales
M-R Scales: Morgan and Russell Scales[171]	Structured interview to give a brief but thorough assessment of the central clinical features of anorexia nervosa; 5 subscales: eating behavior, menstrual state, mental state, relevant attitudes, socioeconomic state; sixth scale allows a self-progress rating.
M-R-H Scale; Morgan-Russell-Hayward Scale[172]	Guided interview concerned with clinical features of anorexia nervosa to evaluate eating behavior, body weight, mental state, and other attitudes relevant to anorexia nervosa; 5 scales: nutrition, menses, mental state, psycho-sexual state, socioeconomic state; additional subscales include: food intake, concern at body image, body weight, menstrual pattern, disturbance of mental state, attitudes toward sexual matters, overt sexual behavior, attitude to menstruation, relationship with family, emancipation from family, personal contacts, social activities, employment record.
MRT: Vandenberg and Kuse's Adaptation of Shepard and Metzler's Three-dimensional Mental Rotations Test[173]	Self-report test of visuospatial ability in which participants view a depiction of a 3-dimensional target figure and 4 test figures and determine which of the test figures are rotated versions of the target figure.
PARQ: Parent Adolescent Relationship Questionnaire[174]	Instrument completed by parents and adolescents 10 through 19 years of age to measure relationship between parents and adolescents; 3 scales: Overt Conflict/Skill Deficits, Extreme Beliefs, Family Structure.
PGWB: Dupuy's Psychological General Well-being Index[175]	Self-report inventory to measure self-representations of intrapersonal affective or emotional states reflecting a sense of subjective well-being or distress; 6 intrapersonal subscales: anxiety, depressed mood, positive well-being, self-control, general health, vitality.
PSE: Present State Examination[176]	Global index of mental state disturbance.
PSR: Psychiatric Status Rating[177]	Clinician-administered instrument to determine the severity of a range of psychiatric disorders that has been used to determine eating disorder outcomes.
QEWP-R: Questionnaire of Eating and Weight Patterns – Revised[178]	Self-report questionnaire to assess a range of features and problems associated with obesity and eating disorders.
RAS: Rathus Assertiveness Schedule[179]	Self-report instrument to measure assertiveness.
RSE: Rosenberg Self-Esteem Scale[180]	Self-report instrument to measure overall self-esteem.
SADS-C: Schedule for Affective Disorders and Schizophrenia-Change Version[181]	Structured interview to differentiate schizophrenia from mood disorders; 2 subscales: depression, mania.
SAMS (Situational Appetite Measures) Urge and SAMS Efficacy[182]	Complementary scales to measure the strength of the urge to binge in 40 different situations and the degree of confidence in one's ability to resist a binge in those same 40 situations.
SAS: Social Adjustment Scale[183]	Self-report questionnaire to assess social and work-related functions; 6 subscales: work, social and leisure, extended family, marital, prenatal, family unit.
SCFI: Standardized Clinical Family Interview[184]	Standardized clinical interview used with families in which the interviewer tries to get responses from all family members and adopts a neutral style. Questions concern numerous areas of family life, mainly what sort of family it is, who does what, who is like whom, life cycle, roles and responsibilities, conflicts, decisions, discipline, relation to the environment.
SCI: Shapiro Control Inventory[185]	Self-report measure of the psychological construct of control (comparable to Locus of Control scales) with 9 subscales.

Table 5. Diagnostic and outcome measures used in randomized controlled trials and outcome studies (continued)

Acronym and Full Name of Test	Description of Test and Subscales
SCID-I: Structured Clinical Interview I for the DSM IV[186]	Structured diagnostic interview to assess presence of current or past DSM IV Axis I major psychiatric disorders.
SCL-90 R Symptom Checklist 90-Revised[134]	General measure of psychopathology, including various forms of anxiety, depression, paranoia, psychotic features. Subscales: Global Severity Index (GSI) to measure overall psychological distress; Positive Symptom Distress Index to measure the intensity of symptoms; Positive Symptom Total of number of self-reported symptoms (Somatization, Obsessive-Compulsive, Interpersonal Sensitivity, Depression, Hostility, Phobic Anxiety, Paranoid Ideation, Psychoticism).
SDS: Zung Self-rating Depression Scale[187]	Self-report assessment to quantify depression, using criteria of pervasive depressed affect and its physiological and psychological concomitants.
SF-36: Medical Outcomes Study Short Form Health Survey[188]	Self-report questionnaire to assess health-related quality of life; 8 subscales: physical function, role physical, bodily pain, general health, mental health, role emotional, social function, vitality, 2 composite scores: physical health; mental health.
SIAB-P: Structured Interview for Anorexia and Bulimia Nervosa[189]	Interview to assess severity of current eating disorder symptoms; 6 subscales: body image and ideal of slimness, social integration and sexuality, depression, obsessive compulsive syndromes and anxiety, bulimic symptoms, laxative abuse.
SMFQ: Short Mood and Feeling Questionnaire[190]	Self-report measure of childhood and adolescent depression for children 8 to 16 years of age.
SOC: Stages of Change Scale[191]	Self-report inventory to describe how respondents feel as they initiate counseling; 4 subscales: Precontemplation, Contemplation, Action, Maintenance.
SPAQ: Seasonal Patterns Assessment Questionnaire[192]	Self-report instrument to rate the presence and severity of seasonal variation in mood, sleep, and eating-related variables; 2 added items monitor seasonal bingeing and purging patterns.
STAI: State Trait Anxiety Inventory[193]	Standardized self-report assessment of both state and trait anxiety (2 subscales).
STAXI: State Trait Anger Expression Inventory[194]	Self-report inventory to assess components of anger and anger expression of normal and abnormal personality.
STPI: State Trait Personality Inventory[193]	Self-report personality inventory.
SUDS: Subjective Units of Distress[195]	Self-report measure of intensity of subjective distress in response to a particular stimulus.
TAS-20: Toronto Alexithymia Scale[196]	Self-report inventory to assess the alexithymia construct (difficulty recognizing, identifying, and communicating emotions; reduced fantasy capacity; and an externally oriented cognitive style); 2 dimensions: identifying feelings (DIF), describing feelings (DDF).
TCI: Temperament and Character Inventory[197]	Self-report measure of temperament and character; 7 subscales: Novelty Seeking, Harm Avoidance, Reward Dependence, Persistence, Self-Directedness, Cooperativeness, Self-Transcendence.
TFEQ: Three-Factor Eating Questionnaire[198]	Self-report inventory; 3 subscales: Cognitive-Restraint, Hunger, Disinhibition. Also known as the Eating Inventory.
WAIS: Wechsler Adult Intelligence Scale[199]	Structured, clinician-administered general test of intelligence for persons 16 years of age and older; 6 Verbal tests: Information, Comprehension, Arithmetic, Digit Span, Similarities, Vocabulary; 5 Performance subtests: Picture Arrangement, Picture Completion, Block Design, Object Assembly, Digit Symbol.
WELSQ: Weight Efficacy Life Style Questionnaire[200]	Self-report measure of confidence about successfully resisting the desire to eat; 5 situational subscales: Negative Emotions, Availability, Social Pressure, Physical Discomfort, Positive Activities.

Table 5. Diagnostic and outcome measures used in randomized controlled trials and outcome studies (continued)

Acronym and Full Name of Test	Description of Test and Subscales
WLFL: Work, Leisure and Family Life Questionnaire[201]	Self-report instrument to measure social adjustment and functioning; 8 scales: work outside the home, housework, social and leisure activities, extended family, marital, parental-older children, parental-baby, family unit.
YBC-EDS and YBOCS-ED: Yale-Brown-Cornell Eating Disorder Scale[202]	Interview to assess preoccupations and rituals associated with eating disorders: symptom checklist produces 3 dimensions of preoccupations and rituals (severity, motivation, ego syntonicity) and covers 18 general categories of rituals and preoccupations.
Y-BOCS- BE: Yale-Brown Obsessive Compulsive Scale Modified for Binge Eating[203]	Clinician-rated inventory of obsessive-compulsive problems adapted for use with binge-eating disorder.
Y-BOCS Score: Yale-Brown Obsessive Compulsive Scale[204]	Clinician-rated scale with separate subtotals for severity of obsessions and compulsions; 2 subscales: obsessions, compulsions.
Youth Self-Report[139,205]	Self-report inventory on various behavior problems.

Chapter 3. Results: Anorexia Nervosa

This chapter presents results of our literature search and our findings for the key questions (KQs) regarding treatment for anorexia nervosa (AN). We examine evidence for the efficacy of various treatments or combinations of treatments for AN (KQ 1), harms associated with the treatment or combination of treatments for AN (KQ 2), factors associated with the efficacy of treatment for AN (KQ 3), and whether the efficacy of treatment for AN differs by sex, gender, age, race, ethnicity, or cultural groups (KQ 4).

We report first on specific details about the yields of the literature searches and characteristics of the studies, then on literature pertaining to treatment (KQs 1 to 4). For each included study, detailed evidence tables appear in Appendix C.[*] We report first on medication trials (Evidence Table 1), then combined medication and behavioral interventions (Evidence Table 2), then behavioral interventions separately for adults (Evidence Table 3), and adolescents (Evidence Table 4). We distinguish between behavioral interventions for adolescents and adults in order to address age differences (KQ 4) as clearly as possible, given the current state of the literature. Within each evidence table, studies are listed alphabetically by author.

Overview of Included Studies

We identified 32 studies published in 35 articles addressing treatment efficacy for AN; of these 15 were medication trials. We were unable to categorize medication studies into adolescent and adult trials given the paucity of medication trials focusing on adolescents.

We rated two medication trials as good,[206] six as fair,[207-213] and seven as poor (not discussed further).[124,214-219] Of the studies judged fair or good, the medications studied included second-generation antidepressants,[206,207] tricyclic antidepressants,[208,209] nutritional supplements,[213] and hormones.[210-212] Study designs included medication versus placebo (six trials), medication A versus medication B versus placebo (one), and medication versus waiting list or nonmedication control (one).

Eighteen of the 32 studies were behavioral intervention trials. In this report behavioral interventions refer to all forms of psychotherapy including cognitive, supportive, dynamic, family, individual, and group. One trial was of therapeutic warming.[220] We rated two of these trials as good,[221,222] nine as fair,[223-231] and six as poor (not discussed further).[220,232-236] Of the 11 trials reviewed here, six were conducted among adults and five among adolescents. Behavioral interventions studied include cognitive behavioral therapy (CBT),[223-225] cognitive analytic therapy (CAT),[226] focal psychoanalytic therapy,[228] and various forms of family therapy.[221,222,229-231,237] The behavioral intervention trials used two designs: psychotherapy A versus psychotherapy B, and psychotherapy A versus psychotherapy B versus control.

We do not discuss studies with a quality rating of "poor" further; reasons these studies received this rating are presented in Table 6. While studies were not lacking in all areas, the most frequent deficiencies across studies contributing to a poor rating include the following: a fatal flaw in the approach to randomization or the approach not being described; investigators and outcome assessors not being blinded to study arm or their blinding status not being described; adverse events not being reported; the statistical analysis not including or not reporting whether a power analysis was conducted; a lack of necessary controls for confounding

---

[*] Appendixes cited in this report are provided electronically at
http://www.ahrq.gov/downloads/pub/evidence/pdf/eatingdisorders/eatdis.pdf.

Table 6. Reasons for poor quality ratings and number of trials with poor ratings: anorexia nervosa

Reasons Contributing to Poor Ratings	Types of Intervention, Number of Times Flaw Was Detected, and Citations
Research Aim	
Hypothesis not clearly described	Medication-only trials: 0
	Behavioral intervention trials (adults): 0
	Behavioral intervention trials (adolescents): 0
Study Population	
Characteristics not clearly described	Medication-only trials: 0
	Behavioral intervention trials (adults): 0
	Behavioral intervention trials (adolescents): 0
No specific inclusion or exclusion criteria	Medication-only trials: 1[214]
	Behavioral intervention trials (adults): 1[233]
	Behavioral intervention trials (adolescents): 0
Randomization	
Protections against influence not in place	Medication-only trials: 6[124,214-216,218,219]
	Behavioral intervention trials (adults): 1[233]
	Behavioral intervention trials (adolescents): 0
Approach not described	Medication-only trial: 6[124,214-216,218,219]
	Behavioral intervention trials (adults): 1[233]
	Behavioral intervention trials (adolescents): 1[236]
Whether randomization had a fatal flaw not known	Medication-only trials: 6[124,214-216,218,219]
	Behavioral intervention trials (adults): 1[233]
	Behavioral intervention trials (adolescents): 2[235,236]
Comparison group(s) not similar at baseline	Medication-only trials: 3[214,215,219]
	Behavioral intervention trials (adults): 0
	Behavioral intervention trials (adolescents): 1[236]
Blinding	
Study subjects	Medication-only trials: 4[215-217,219]
	Behavioral intervention trials (adults): N/A
	Behavioral intervention trials (adolescents): N/A
Investigators	Medication-only trials: 6[124,215-219]
	Behavioral intervention trials (adults): 1[220]
	Behavioral intervention trials (adolescents): 0

N/A, not applicable.

Table 6. Reasons for poor quality ratings and number of trials with poor ratings: anorexia nervosa (continued)

Reasons Contributing to Poor Ratings	Types of Intervention, Number of Times Flaw Was Detected, and Citations
Outcomes assessors	Medication-only trials: 6[124,215-219]
	Behavioral intervention trials (adults): 3[220,233,234]
	Behavioral intervention trials (adolescents): 2[235,236]
Interventions	
Interventions not clearly described	Medication-only trials: 0
	Behavioral intervention trials (adults): 0
	Behavioral intervention trials (adolescents): 0
No reliable measurement of patient compliance	Medication-only trials: 5[214-217,219]
	Behavioral intervention trials (adults): 1[220]
	Behavioral intervention trials (adolescents): 1[235]
Outcomes	
Results not clearly described	Medication-only trials: 0
	Behavioral intervention trials (adults): 2[220,233]
	Behavioral intervention trials (adolescents): 0
Adverse events not reported	Medication-only trials: 3[214,215,217]
	Behavioral intervention trials (adults): 2[233,234]
	Behavioral intervention trials (adolescents): 1[235]
Statistical Analysis	
Statistics inappropriate	Medication-only trials: 0
	Behavioral intervention trials (adults): 3[220,232,233]
	Behavioral intervention trials (adolescents): 0
No controls for confounding (if needed)	Medication-only trials: 3[214,218,219]
	Behavioral intervention trials (adults): 2[232,233]
	Behavioral intervention trials (adolescents): 2[235,236]
Intention-to-treat analysis not used	Medication-only trials: 5[214,215,217-219]
	Behavioral intervention trials (adults): 2[220,233]
	Behavioral intervention trials (adolescents): 2[235,236]
Power analysis not done or not reported	Medication-only trials: 7[124,214-219]
	Behavioral intervention trials (adults): 4[220,232-234]
	Behavioral intervention trials (adolescents): 1[235]

Table 6. Reasons for poor quality ratings and number of trials with poor ratings: anorexia nervosa (continued)

Reasons Contributing to Poor Ratings	Types of Intervention, Number of Times Flaw Was Detected, and Citations
Results	
Loss to followup 26% or higher or not reported	Medication-only trials: 2[214,215]
	Behavioral intervention trials (adults): 1[233]
	Behavioral intervention trials (adolescents): 0
Differential loss to followup 15% or higher or not reported	Medication-only trials: 1[214,215]
	Behavioral intervention trials (adults): 3[220,233,234]
	Behavioral intervention trials (adolescents): 1[236]
Outcome measures not standard, reliable, or valid in all groups	Medication-only trials: 0
	Behavioral intervention trials (adults): 1[220]
	Behavioral intervention trials (adolescents): 0
Discussion	
Results do not support conclusions, taking possible biases and limitations into account	Medication-only trials: 0
	Behavioral intervention trials (adults): 0
	Behavioral intervention trials (adolescents): 0
Results not discussed within context of prior research	Medication-only trials: 0
	Behavioral intervention trials (adults): 0
External validity: population not representative of US population relevant to these treatments	Medication-only trials: 3[215,217,218]
	Behavioral intervention trials (adults): 1[220]
	Behavioral intervention trials (adolescents): 0
Funding/sponsorship not reported	Medication-only trials: 6[214-219]
	Behavioral intervention trials (adults): 3[220,232,234]
	Behavioral intervention trials (adolescents): 1[235]

or results not presented using an intention-to-treat approach; and sources of funding not being stated.

Dropouts are a significant element in the quality of all these trials. Table 7 documents the total sample size and attrition rates in the trials reviewed in this chapter.

Participants

Of the 19 studies rated fair or good, 10 were conducted in the United States, six in the United Kingdom, two in Canada, and one in New Zealand. A total of 891 individuals participated in fair or good clinical trials for AN. One study failed to report sex. From those studies that reported sex, 861 women and 23 men participated. Seventeen studies failed to report ethnicity for participants. Of those that did, 123 participants were identified as white, eight as Asian and three as other ethnicity.

Table 7. Dropout rates for randomized controlled trials: anorexia nervosa

Author	Total Enrollment	Total Dropouts	Group 1 Treatment (% dropout)	G2 Treatment (% dropout)	G3 Treatment (% dropout)	G4 Treatment (% dropout)
			Medication Trials			
Attia et al., 1998[206]	33	1 (+1 unreliable self-reporter) (3%)	Fluoxetine (NR)	Placebo (NR)		
Kaye et al., 2001[207]	39	26 (66%)	Fluoxetine (16% at 30 days, 47% at 1 year)	Placebo (5% at 30 days, 85% at 1 year)		
Biederman et al.,1985[209]	25	0 (0%)	Amitriptyline (0%)	Placebo (0%)		
Halmi et al.,1986[208]	72	18 (25%)	Amitriptyline (30%)	Cyproheptadine (25%)	Placebo (20%)	
Hill, et al., 2000[212]	15	0 (0%)	Recombinant human growth hormone (0%)	Placebo (0%)		
Klibanski et al., 1995[210]	48	4 (8%)	Estrogen/ progestin (14%)	Control (4%)		
Miller, Grieco, and Klibanski 2005[211]	38	5 (13%)	Testosterone (NR)	Placebo (NR)		
Birmingham, Goldner, and Bakan1994[213]	54	19 (35%)	Zinc (39%)	Placebo (32%)		
			Behavioral Intervention Trials (Adult)			
Channon et al., 1989[225]	24	3 (13%)	CBT (0%)	Behavioral treatment (13%)	Control (25%)	
McIntosh et al., 2005[224]	56	21 (38%)	CBT (37%)	Interpersonal psychotherapy (43%)	Nonspecific supportive clinical management (31%)	
Pike et al., 2003[223]	33	3 (9%)	CBT (0%)	Nutritional counseling (20%)		
Dare et al., 2001[228]	84	30 (36%)	Focal psychotherapy (43%)	Family therapy (27%)	Cognitive analytic therapy (41%)	Routine (32%)
Treasure et al., 1995[226]	30	10 (33%)	Educational behavioral therapy (38%)	Cognitive analytic therapy (29%)		
Crisp et al., 1991[227] and Gowers et al.,1994[238]	90	17 (19%)	Inpatient (40%)	Outpatient psychotherapy/ family therapy/ dietary counseling (10%)	Group therapy (15%)	No further treatment (0%)

CBT, cognitive behavioral therapy; NR, not reported.

Author	Total Enrollment	Total Dropouts	Group 1 Treatment (% dropout)	G2 Treatment (% dropout)	G3 Treatment (% dropout)	G4 Treatment (% dropout)
		Behavioral Intervention Trials (Adolescent)				
Eisler et al., 2000[221]	40	4 (10%)	Conjoint family therapy (11%)	Separated family therapy (10%)		
Geist et al., 2000[229]	25	0 (0%)	Family therapy (0%)	Family group psychoeducation (0%)		
Russell et al., 1987[231] and Eisler et al., 1997[239]	80	28 (35%)	Family therapy (37%)	Individual therapy (33%)		
Robin et al., 1994[230] and Robin, Siegel, and Moye 1995[237]	24	2 (8%)	Behavioral family systems therapy (8%)	Ego-oriented individual therapy (8%)		
Lock et al., 2005[222]	86	17 (20%)	Long-term treatment (24%)	Short-term treatment (16%)		

Key Question 1: Treatment Efficacy

Medication Trials

Table 8 presents results from medication treatment trials for AN, including treatment aims, setting (inpatient or outpatient), and a summary of outcomes. Similar to text, it is organized by medication class. Of the identified AN trials, eight were randomized controlled double-blind medication trials. Medication trials for AN were most commonly conducted in the context of clinical management or during or following inpatient refeeding. Of these, none reported race or ethnicity of participants, while all but one reported sex of participants; six were conducted in the United States. One study explicitly reported intention-to-treat analyses.[212] The number of participants in the medication trials ranged from 15 to 72, with the total enrollment for all medication trials being 345. Thus, the average number of patients per study was 23. Based on those studies that reported sex, this includes 319 women and 1 man.

Weight gain is the primary outcome variable in the treatment of AN. Secondary outcomes in this population include reduction of the psychological features of AN (e.g., body dissatisfaction and drive for thinness), reduction of associated behaviors such as overexercising, resumption of menses, and, in the bingeing and purging subtype, decreased binge eating and purging behaviors. Additional psychiatric outcomes include reduction in depression and anxiety.

Second-generation antidepressants. The term "second-generation antidepressants" is commonly used in the psychiatric and pharmacological literature to distinguish newer antidepressants such as selective norepinephrine reuptake inhibitors (SNRIs), selective serotonin reuptake inhibitors (SSRIs), bupropion, nefazodone, and trazodone from traditional or first-generation antidepressants such as tricyclic antidepressants and monoamine oxidase inhibitors. We adopted this term to be consistent in terminology with other research conducted in the area of psychopharmacology.

Table 8. Results from medication trials: anorexia nervosa

Source, Treatment, Setting, and Quality Score	Major Outcome Measures	Significant Change Over Time Within Groups	Significant Differences Between Groups at Endpoint	Significant Differences Between Groups in Change Over Time
Attia et al., 1998[206] Fluoxetine vs. placebo Inpatient Good	Eating: • AN behavior • BSQ • CGI • EAT • YBC-EDS Biomarker: • IBW Psych: • BDI • CGI • SCL-90	Both groups experienced decreased clinician-rated ED symptoms and illness severity, ED concerns, depressed mood, obsessive-compulsive symptoms, and food preoccupation and rituals. Both groups increased percent IBW.	No statistics reported.	No differences on any measures.
Kaye et al., 2001[207] Fluoxetine vs. placebo Inpatient and outpatient Fair	Eating: • YBC-EDS Biomarker: • ABW Psych: • HAM-A • HDRS • YBOCS	Fluoxetine completers experienced decreased anxious and depressed mood and increased percent ABW	No differences on any measures.	No differences on any measures.
Biederman et al., 1985[209] Amitriptyline vs. placebo Inpatient and outpatient Fair	Eating: • EAT Biomarker: • Weight Psych: • Global severity • HSCL • SADS-C	No statistics reported.	No differences on any measures.	No statistics reported.

ABW, average body weight; AN, anorexia nervosa; BDI, Beck Depression Inventory; BMI, body mass index; BN, bulimia nervosa; BSQ, Body Shape Questionnaire; CGI, Clinical Global Impressions; EAT, Eating Attitudes Test; ED, eating disorders; HAM-A, Hamilton Anxiety Inventory; HAM-D, Hamilton Depression Inventory; HDRS, Hamilton Depression Rating Scale; HSCL, Hopkins Symptom Checklist; IBW, ideal body weight; Psych, psychiatric and psychological; *rhGH*, recombinant human grown hormone; SADS-C, Schedule for Affective Disorders and Schizophrenia-Change Version; SCL-90, (Hopkins) Symptom Checklist; tx, treatment; vs., versus; YBC-EDS, Yale-Brown-Cornell Eating Disorders Scale; YBOCS, Yale-Brown Obsessive-Compulsive scale.

Table 8. Results from medication trials: anorexia nervosa (continued)

Source, Treatment, Setting, and Quality Score	Major Outcome Measures	Significant Change Over Time Within Groups	Significant Differences Between Groups at Endpoint	Significant Differences Between Groups in Change Over Time
Halmi et al., 1986[208] Amitriptyline vs. cyproheptadine vs. placebo Inpatient Fair	Eating: • Caloric intake Biomarker: • Weight Psych: • HAM-D • BDI • SCL-90	No statistics reported.	Cyproheptadine associated with fewer days to target weight, higher caloric intake, and less depressed mood compared to placebo. BN subgroup: amitriptyline associated with improved tx efficacy compared to cyproheptadine; neither drug differed from placebo. For non-BN subgroup: cyproheptadine associated with improved tx efficacy compared to placebo. No other subgroup comparisons were significant.	No statistics reported.
Hill et al., 2000[212] rhGH vs. placebo Inpatient Good	Biomarker: • Orthostasis • Weight	No statistics reported.	rhGH associated with fewer days to restoration of normal orthostatic response compared to placebo.	No statistics reported.
Klibanski et al., 1995[210] Estrogen/ progestin vs. nonmedication control Outpatient Fair	Eating: • Recovery • Remission Biomarker: • Bone density • Percent Body fat • Percent IBW • Weight	No statistics reported.	No differences on any measures.	No differences on any measures.
Miller et al., 2005[211] Testosterone vs. placebo Setting unknown Fair	Biomarker: • BMI • IBW Psych: • BDI	No statistics reported.	Testosterone associated with less depressed mood compared to placebo.	Depressed mood increased less in testosterone-treated group.
Birmingham et al., 1994[213] Zinc vs. placebo Inpatient Fair	Biomarker: • BMI • Percent body fat • Weight	No statistics reported.	No differences on any measures.	Zinc superior to placebo in rate of BMI increase.

Fluoxetine. Two trials used fluoxetine at different stages of refeeding in AN patients. In an inpatient study, Attia et al.[206] randomized 31 females between 16 and 45 years who had achieved weight restoration of at least 65 percent of ideal body weight (IBW) to fluoxetine (60 mg/day) or placebo. The mean BMI at randomization was 15 kg/m^2. Patients continued to receive psychotherapy. No significant differences emerged between fluoxetine and placebo on weight gain (16 versus 13 pounds), psychological features of eating disorders, or depression or anxiety measures. Three percent of participants dropped out of fluoxetine treatment.

In the second study, patients were randomly assigned to either initiation on fluoxetine or placebo before inpatient discharge with a beginning dosage of 20 mg/day adjusted over 52 weeks to a maximum of 60 mg/day.[207] The range of weight for all participants at randomization was 76 percent to 100 percent average body weight (ABW) with the majority above 90 percent. Outpatient psychotherapy was permitted. Dropout was considerable. Of 39 individuals randomized, only 13 remained at the 52-week endpoint (47 percent of fluoxetine and 85 percent of placebo). In this small group of completers, fluoxetine was associated with significantly greater weight gain, reduced anxiety, depression, obsessive-compulsive features, and eating-disorder-related symptoms.

Tricyclic antidepressants. Two trials of fair or good quality investigated tricyclic antidepressant medication use. Neither provided strong data supporting the use of these medications in treating AN patients.

Amitriptyline in doses up to 175 mg/day in 25 youth ages 11 to 17 years led to no significant differences in eating, mood, or weight outcomes in comparison to placebo.[209] No patients dropped out in this trial. Halmi et al. compared amitriptyline (160 mg/day) versus cyproheptadine (32 mg/day) versus placebo in 72 females 13 to 36 years, determined to have AN according to the Diagnostic and Statistical Manual, third edition (DSM III).[208] Daily caloric intake was significantly higher in cyproheptadine than placebo and significantly fewer days were needed to achieve target weight (in those who did) in both the amitriptyline and cyproheptadine groups, compared with placebo. Drop out was thirty percent in the amitriptyline group, 25 percent in the cyproheptadine group, and 20 percent in the placebo group.

Hormones. Investigators have studied three hormones in the treatment of AN: growth hormone (rGH), testosterone, and estrogen. Three weeks of transdermal testosterone (150 mg or 330 mg) administered to 38 patients with AN ages 18 to 50 led to greater decreases in depression in patients who were depressed at baseline, but differences in weight were not interpretable.[211] Dropout was 13 percent overall.

Growth hormone (15 mg/kg/day) administered to 14 female and 1 male patient receiving inpatient care for AN led to fewer days to display normal orthostatic heart rate response to a standing challenge among the treatment group than among placebo group.[212] No patient dropped out of this study.

Klibanski et al. compared estrogen/progesterone (0.625 mg Premarin® or 5 mg Provera® per day) versus nonmedication control in 48 females 16 to 43 years and found no differences between groups on bone density at 6 months.[210] Dropout was 14 percent in hormone group and 4 percent in the nonmedication group.

Hormone treatment during the acute phase of AN illness does not appear to improve bone density.[210] Scant, preliminary evidence suggests that rGH leads to faster normalization of orthostatic changes seen in AN[212] and that testosterone improves depression in individuals with AN and depressed mood.[211]

Nutritional supplements. The one study of nutritional supplements was performed in 54 female inpatients older than 15 years with 14 mg/day zinc. It provides preliminary evidence that zinc may increase the rate of increase in BMI.[213] Dropout was 39 percent in zinc and 32 percent in placebo, suggesting that conclusions from this study must be viewed with great caution.

Summary of drug trials. All eight studies assessing the efficacy of medication interventions on AN examined weight gain; most reported on eating outcomes and some reported on additional symptom change.

Overall, none of the pharmacological interventions for AN had a significant impact on weight gain. Although tricyclic antidepressants may be associated with greater improvement in secondary mood outcomes, this outcome does not appear to be associated with improved weight gain. No trial has been adequately replicated.

Dropout rates for medication studies for AN are substantial, especially in outpatient trials. Conclusions drawn from studies with such high attrition must be reviewed with extreme caution.

Taken together, the literature regarding medication treatments for AN is sparse and inconclusive. The vast majority of studies had small sample sizes and rarely had adequate statistical power to allow for definitive conclusions. Many studies examined patients who were receiving additional treatments in conjunction with the study medication, including psychological interventions and concurrent pharmacological treatments. Some of these studies examined patients who were in inpatient settings, thus limiting generalizability to outpatient treatment. Only one conducted intention-to-treat analyses; the remaining studies reported completer analyses only. With one exception,[209] no medication trials have focused on adolescent patients. Because followup was limited, assessing longer-term impact of interventions on such outcomes as bone density was impossible. Finally, only one male participated in any of these studies, thereby making it impossible to draw any conclusions about the pharmacological treatment of AN in boys and men.

Behavioral Intervention Trials

Of the 11 behavior trials rated good or fair (Tables 9 and 10), four focused solely on adolescents (mean ages 14 to 15), six focused solely on adults (approximately 18 years and older), and one combined adolescent and adult patients. Of the 11 trials, four were conducted in the United States. We present behavioral interventions for adults with AN in Table 9.

Behavioral interventions for adults with anorexia nervosa. In the psychotherapy trials for adults only and the combined adult and adolescent trials, investigators tested CBT (three trials), various types of nonspecific therapy (three), family therapies (two), CAT (two), dietary counseling (one), interpersonal psychotherapy (IPT) (one), behavioral therapy (BT) (one), and focal analytic therapy (one).

Cognitive behavioral therapy. CBT studies generally used a form of therapy tailored to AN that focused on cognitive and behavioral features associated with the maintenance of eating pathology. Of the three CBT studies, one followed inpatient weight restoration[223] and two were done in the underweight state.[224,225] CBT significantly reduced relapse risk and increased the likelihood of good outcome compared to nutritional counseling based on nutritional education and food exchanges after inpatient weight restoration.[223] Of those receiving CBT, a greater number of individuals with good outcomes were also receiving antidepressant medication.

One study of underweight AN outpatients compared CBT with IPT and nonspecific supportive clinical management (NSCM).[224] IPT in the treatment of AN is based on IPT used for the treatment of depression[240] and BN;[241] it focuses on one of four interpersonal problem areas:

Table 9. Results from behavioral intervention trials in adults: anorexia nervosa

Source, Treatment, Setting, and Quality Score	Major Outcome Measures	Significant Change Over Time Within Groups	Significant Differences Between Groups at Endpoint	Significant Differences Between Groups in Change Over Time
Channon et al., 1989[225] CBT vs. BT vs. 'Usual care' control Outpatient Fair	Eating: • EDI • M-R scale Biomarker: • BMI • M-R scale Psych: • BDI • MOCI • M-R scale	No statistics reported.	At 6-month FU, CBT associated with better psychosexual functioning than BT and BT was associated with greater improvement in menstrual functioning than CBT. At 1-year FU, the BT group scored better than the CBT group on preferred weight. CBT and BT combined were associated with greater improvements on nutritional functioning than the control group. The control group showed greater improvements on drive for thinness than the combined CBT and BT groups.	No statistics reported.
McIntosh et al., 2005[224] CBT vs. IPT vs. NSCM Outpatient Fair	Eating: • EDE • EDI Biomarker: • BMI • Percent body fat • Weight Psych: • GAF • HDRS		Compared to IPT, NSCM associated with higher likelihood of 'good' global outcome.	NSCM superior to IPT in improving global functioning and eating restraint over 20 weeks. NSCM superior to CBT in improving global functioning over 20 weeks. CBT superior to IPT in improving eating restraint over 20 weeks.
Pike et al., 2003[223] CBT vs. nutritional counseling Outpatient Fair	Eating: • Recovery • Relapse • Tx failure • M-R scale	No statistics reported.	Compared to nutrition counseling, CBT associated with lower percentage tx failures, higher percentage 'good' outcome, and longer time (weeks) to relapse.	No statistics reported.

ABW, average body weight; BDI, Beck Depression Inventory; BMI, body mass index; BT, behavioral therapy; CAT, cognitive-analytic therapy; CBT, cognitive behavioral therapy; EBT, educational behavioral therapy; EDE, Eating Disorders Examination; EDI, Eating Disorders Inventory (EDI-2, Garner, 1991); FU, follow-up; GAF, Global Assessment of Functioning [DSM-IV]; HDRS, Hamilton Depression Rating Scale; IBW, ideal body weight; IPT, interpersonal therapy; MOCI, Maudsley Obsessional Compulsive Index; M-R, Morgan and Russell; NSCM, nonspecific supported clinical management, Psych, psychiatric and psychological; pt, patients; Tx, treatment, vs., versus.

47

Table 9. Results from behavioral intervention trials in adults: anorexia nervosa (continued)

Source, Treatment, Setting, and Quality Score	Major Outcome Measures	Significant Change Over Time Within Groups	Significant Differences Between Groups at Endpoint	Significant Differences Between Groups in Change Over Time
Dare et al., 2001[228] CAT vs. focal vs. family vs. 'routine' therapy Outpatient Fair	Eating: • M-R scale • Recovery Biomarker: • BMI • Percent ABW • M-R scale Psych: • M-R scale	No statistics reported.	At 1-year FU, compared to routine tx, focal and family tx associated with higher weight; also, higher percentage of patients in focal and family tx were recovered or significantly improved (i.e., > 85% IBW, no/few menstrual or BN symptoms).	No statistics reported.
Treasure et al., 1995[226] CAT vs. EBT Outpatient Fair	Eating: • M-R scales Biomarker: • BMI • Weight Psych: • M-R scales • Self progress scale	No statistics reported.	Compared to EBT, CAT associated with higher self-rating of improvement.	No statistics reported.
Crisp et al., 1991[227] and Gowers et al., 1994[238] Inpatient tx vs. outpatient individual and family therapy and dietary counseling vs. group therapy vs. no formal tx Inpatient and outpatient Fair	Eating: • M-R scale • Remission Biomarker: • BMI • M-R scale • Weight Psych: • M-R scale	At 1-year FU, global score and menstruation improved in all 4 groups, nutrition score improved in 3 active tx groups, and mental state improved in outpatient family/diet counseling group. At 2-year FU, mental state improved in outpatient family/diet counseling; global score, menstruation, and nutrition improved in groups that received outpatient family/diet counseling and no formal tx.	Compared to 'no formal tx', outpatient family/diet counseling associated with higher weight and BMI at 1- and 2-year FU.	Compared to 'no formal tx,' weight increased more at 1-year FU in all 3 active groups. Weight increased more at 2-year FU in outpatient family/diet counseling compared to 'no formal tx' group.

Table 10. Results from behavioral intervention trials in adolescents only and adolescents and adults combined: anorexia nervosa

Source, Treatment, Setting, and Quality Score	Major Outcome Measures	Significant Change Over Time Within Groups	Significant Differences Between Groups at Endpoint	Significant Differences Between Groups in Change Over Time
Eisler et al., 2000[221] CFT vs. SFT Outpatient Good	Eating: • Bulimic symptoms • EAT • EDI Biomarker: • Percent ABW • BMI • Weight Psych: • MOCI • SMFQ • Depression • Obsessionality	No statistics reported.	No statistics reported.	CFT superior to SFT in reducing ED-related traits, depression, and obsessionality.
Geist et al., 2000[229] Family therapy vs. family group psycho-education Inpatient Fair	Eating: • EDI Biomarker: • Percent IBW Psych: • BSI • CDI • FAM III	No statistics reported.	No differences on any measures.	No differences on any measures.
Russell et al., 1987[231] and Eisler et al., 1997[239] Family therapy vs. individual therapy Outpatient Fair	Eating: • M-R scales • Readmit rate Biomarker: • Percent ABW • M-R scales • Weight Psych: • M-R scales	No statistics reported.	No statistics reported.	Among early onset, less chronic AN patients, family therapy superior to individual therapy in improving nutritional status, menstrual and psychosexual function, and weight over 1 year tx; family therapy also more likely associated with a 'good' outcome over 1-year tx and 5-year FU.

ABW, average body weight; AN, anorexia nervosa; BDI, Beck Depression Inventory; BFST, behavioral family systems therapy; BMI, body mass index; BSI, Brief Symptom Inventory; BSQ, Body Shape Questionnaire; CDI, Children's Depression Inventory; CFT, conjoint family therapy; EAT, Eating Attitudes Test; ED, eating disorders; EDE, Eating Disorders Examination; EDI, Eating Disorders Inventory; EOIT, ego-oriented individual therapy; FAM-III, Family Assessment Measure; FU, follow-up; IBC, Interaction Behavior Code; IBW, ideal body weight; MOCI, Maudsley Obsessional Compulsive Index; M-R, Morgan and Russell; PARQ, Parent Adolescent Relationship Questionnaire; Psych, psychiatric and psychological; SFT, separated family therapy; SMFQ, Short Mood and Feeling Questionnaire; tx, treatment; vs., versus; YBC-EDS, Yale-Brown-Cornell Eating Disorders Scale.

Table 10. Results from behavioral intervention trials in adolescents only and adolescents combined: anorexia nervosa (continued)

Source, Treatment, Setting, and Quality Score	Major Outcome Measures	Significant Change Over Time Within Groups	Significant Differences Between Groups at Endpoint	Significant Differences Between Groups in Change Over Time
Robin et al., 1994[230] and Robin et al., 1995[237] BFST vs. EOIT Outpatient and inpatient Fair	Eating: • EAT • EDI • Eating conflict Biomarker: • BMI • Weight • Menstruation Psych: • BDI • BSQ • PARQ • IBC	No statistics reported.	No differences on any measures.	BFST superior to EOIT in increasing BMI to post-tx and 1-year FU, and in improving mother's positive communication at FU.
Lock et al., 2005[222] Long-term vs. short-term family therapy Outpatient Good	Eating: • EDE • YBC-EDS Biomarker: • BMI • Weight	No differences on any measures.	No differences on any measures.	No differences on any measures among those with most severe YBC-EDS symptoms. Longer-term tx associated with better BMI outcome in those with most severe ED symptoms, and with better EDE global outcome in those with non-intact families.

interpersonal disputes, role transitions, grief, or interpersonal deficits. NSCM was designed for this study to mimic the type of treatment an individual could receive in the community from a provider familiar with the treatment of ED and incorporates elements of sound clinical management and supportive psychotherapy. In an intention-to-treat analysis, NSCM performed significantly better than IPT in producing global good outcome ratings; CBT outcomes fell in between and were not significantly different from the other two outcomes.[224] The second study compared CBT with BT and a control group for 6 months.[225] At 12-month followup, CBT showed no advantage over BT or control in eating, mood, or weight outcomes.

On the basis of one trial, preliminary evidence suggests that CBT delivered after weight restoration may help to decrease relapse. In contrast, when delivered during the acute phase of the illness, CBT does not appear to offer significant advantage over NSCM, which did offer advantage over IPT. No evidence suggests that nutritional counseling alone is efficacious in the treatment of AN.

Cognitive analytic therapy (CAT). The two studies that utilized CAT, a treatment which integrates psychodynamic with behavioral factors and focuses on interpersonal and transference issues, failed to find any advantage of CAT over educational behavioral therapy or focal family therapy in eating, mood, or weight outcomes.[226,228] Focal family therapy focused on eliminating the eating disorder from its controlling role in determining the relationship between the patient and other family members.

Family therapy. Of the three studies in this category, Dare et al. found family therapy to be superior to routine treatment but equivalent to a focal time-limited psychodynamic psychotherapy in increasing percentage of adult body weight, restoring menstruation, and decreasing bulimic symptoms; overall clinical improvement was modest, however.[228]

Crisp et al.[227] found outpatient individual and family therapy with variable numbers of sessions to be superior to referral to a family physician for increased weight at 1- and 2-year followup.

The efficacy of family therapy in treating adults with AN has not yet been completely addressed. It may be more effective than medical management by a family physician and routine treatment; family therapy (including the family of origin) may be more effective in younger patients with shorter duration of illness. No studies have explored family therapy for adult patients that included the family of insertion (spouse and offspring of the patient) rather than the family of origin.

Behavioral interventions for adolescents with anorexia nervosa. We present behavioral interventions for adolescents with AN in Table 10.

Family therapy. Four family therapy studies focused exclusively on adolescents and one combined adolescent and adult patients.[231] Family therapy was more effective for younger patients with earlier onset than for older patients with a more chronic course in the United Kingdom trial performed by Russell et al.[231] and the followup by Eisler et al.[239] These studies did not yield evidence that the specific type of family therapy administered was helpful for the older more chronic group.[228,231] A form of family therapy focusing initially on parental control of re-nutrition delivered in two different manners revealed a significant advantage of conjoint therapy (family treated as a unit) over separated family therapy (parents and patient seen separately) on eating and mood outcomes but not on weight outcomes.[221]

In a second study, no differences emerged between family therapy and family psychoeducation on any outcomes at 16 weeks.[229] For a specific form of family therapy, when delivered in conjunction with a common medical and dietary regimen, behavioral family systems therapy (BFST), also characterized initially by parents taking control of renutrition, Robin et al. found BFST to be superior to ego-oriented individual therapy in increasing BMI and restoring menstruation, although neither therapy was superior on eating or mood outcomes.[230,237] Addressing the issue of optimal duration of family therapy, Lock et al. randomized adolescents to either short (10 sessions over 6 months) or long (20 sessions over 12 months) manualized family therapy based on the initial parental control of refeeding model[242] and found no differences on eating, psychiatric, or biomarker outcomes.[222] Longer-term family therapy suggested that those with more severe eating-related obsessions and nonintact families did better with longer treatment. Finally, in the one study that included both adolescents and adults, family therapy was superior to individual therapy for adolescent patients with shorter duration of illness. This difference did not emerge for adult patients with longer duration of illness.[231] Although few differences were observed across interventions, specific forms of family interventions did consistently show improvement over time with adolescent patients.

Summary of behavioral interventions for adults and adolescents with anorexia nervosa. Overall, one study of adults provides tentative evidence that CBT may reduce relapse risk for adults with AN after weight restoration has been accomplished.[223] Sufficient evidence does not exist to determine whether CBT is effective during the acute phase of the illness (i.e., in the underweight state before weight restoration); one study found that a manualized nonspecific supportive treatment (NCSM) was more effective than CBT or IPT in terms of global outcome during the acute phase.[224] The three family therapy studies provide no support for the efficacy of the type of family therapy delivered in adults with AN with longer duration of illness; the superiority of this approach for younger patients with a shorter illness course is based on one study.[231] Two studies failed to find any benefit of CAT for eating, mood, or weight outcomes when compared to other treatments for this population.[226,228] No methodologically sound studies that systematically tested combinations of medication and psychotherapy were identified.

Serious methodological concerns arose with some of these trials. Two were very small (8 to 12 participants per group),[225,230] which does not provide adequate statistical power for the comparative analyses conducted. In addition, both had marked pretreatment differences between groups. Failure to control for contact time with a clinician while comparing multiple treatments, with some groups getting up to 80 percent more time in treatment than others, was another problem.[228] In addition, only one group of researchers conducted a follow-up study to determine the long-term impact of their interventions.[239]

Five studies evaluated family therapy in adolescents with AN. Overall, family therapy based on principles of parental control of initial refeeding leads to clinically meaningful weight gain and psychological change. However, the majority of family therapy studies compares one form of family therapy to another form and were underpowered to detect significant differences between active similar treatments. One study suggested that family therapy was superior to a non-family therapy comparison intervention for adolescent patients with relatively short duration of illness.[231] One additional study reported significantly greater weight gain at the end of treatment in family therapy than in ego-oriented individual therapy for adolescent AN patients.[230] The other three studies all involved some sort of family treatment – either comparing conjoint to separated family therapy or comparing family therapy to family psychoeducation.[221,229] Conjoint therapy was superior to separated family therapy for improving eating and mood but not weight outcomes.[221] Similarly, one study examining family therapy versus family psychoeducation found no differences between groups.[229]

Inadequate statistical power was a common problem among the behavioral interventions in AN, and power calculations were rarely reported. No studies had a pure no-treatment condition, which is appropriate given the gravity of the illness, although "usual" treatment took various forms. Many of these studies had adequate power to detect pre-post within-group differences or differences between no treatment and an active treatment, but few were adequately powered to detect differences across two or more treatment groups.

Key Question 2: Harms of Treatment for Anorexia Nervosa

Table 11 presents adverse events associated with treatments for AN reported in each of the 32 studies reviewed. Assuming that all relevant adverse events were reported, the most common was the need for inpatient treatment among participants in an outpatient trial. Eight studies reported that one or more participants dropped out because of the need for inpatient treatment. In one study, a participant died before commencing the intervention. In these cases, the events observed may be more ongoing features of the course of illness than an adverse event caused by the intervention per se. In behavioral interventions, physical and psychological harms of interventions are rarely reported.

For the trials using second-generation antidepressants, we refer to recent publications on the comparative effectiveness and tolerability of second-generation antidepressants.[243] Common side

Table 11. Adverse events reported: anorexia nervosa

Intervention	Adverse Events Reported*
Medication Trials	
Fluoxetine vs. placebo[206]	Fluoxetine group: insomnia and agitation; blurred vision
Fluoxetine vs. placebo[207]	No adverse events observed
Amitriptyline vs. cyproheptadine vs. placebo[208]	Amitriptyline: drowsiness, excitement, confusion, increased motor activity, tachycardia, dry mouth, constipation. Cyproheptadine: no consistent pattern observed Placebo: drowsiness, excitement, increased motor activity.
Amitriptyline vs. placebo[209]	Amitriptyline group: diaphoresis (2), drowsiness (6), dry mouth (4), blurred vision (1), urinary retention (1), hypotension (2), leucopenia (1) Placebo: dry mouth (2), palpitations (1), dizziness (2)
Estrogen vs. nonmedication control[210]	Estrogen group: depression (1), hyperlipidemia (1)
Growth hormone vs. placebo[212]	No adverse events observed
Testosterone vs. placebo[211]	Testosterone group: Mild skin irritation at patch site (3), increased depression (1), increased fatigue and vertigo (1), nausea (1) Placebo: Mild skin irritation at patch site (1)
Zinc vs. placebo[213]	NR
Behavioral Interventions Trials	
Behavioral family systems vs. ego-oriented individual[230,237]	NR
CBT vs. behavioral therapy vs. control[225]	NR
CBT vs. interpersonal psychotherapy vs. nonspecific supportive clinical management[224]	No adverse events observed
CBT vs. nutritional counseling[223]	CBT: Depression and suicidal ideation (1) Nutritional: Depression and suicidal ideation (3)
Cognitive analytical vs. educational behavioral[226]	NR
Conjoint family vs. separated family[221]	NR
Family therapy vs. family group psychoeducation[229]	NR
Family therapy vs. nonspecific individual[231,239]	NR
Focal psychotherapy vs. family therapy vs. cognitive analytical vs. routine treatment[228]	NR
Inpatient + 12 individual/family vs. outpatient individual/family variable vs. 10 outpatient group vs. family physician vs. dietary counseling[227,238]	NR
Short- vs. long-term family therapy[222]	NR: Dropout attributed to other psychological problems

CBT, cognitive behavioral therapy; NR, not reported; vs., versus.
* If no numbers appear in parentheses, authors had only listed adverse events but not reported the number of cases.

effects associated with the use of second-generation antidepressants in major depressive disorder are nausea, headache, diarrhea, constipation, dizziness, fatigue, sweating, and sexual side effects. Rare but severe adverse events include hyponatremia, suicidality, and seizures. Up to 90 percent of patients experienced at least one adverse event during treatment. Overall, discontinuation rates attributed to adverse events did not differ significantly among individual drugs and ranged from 6 percent to 14 percent. The authors report no substantial differences in adverse events with respect to drugs that were also used in eating disorders trials (i.e., citalopram, fluoxetine, fluvoxamine, and sertraline).

Given the small sample sizes and completion rates of the two fluoxetine trials, we cannot draw definitive conclusions regarding whether harms associated with fluoxetine treatment in the underweight state differ in any way from treatment of normal-weight individuals with other psychiatric diagnoses. In these studies, Kaye et al. failed to report adverse events;[207] Attia et al. reported one case of insomnia and agitation and one case of blurred vision.[206]

For tricyclic antidepressants, Halmi et al. reported sporadic cases of drowsiness, excitement, confusion, increased motor activity, tachycardia, dry mouth, and constipation associated with amitriptyline;[208] however, the rate of adverse events did not differ from placebo.

The only specific adverse event associated with testosterone administration was skin irritation at the patch site. Estrogen administration yielded one case of depression and one of hyperlipidemia. No adverse effects were reported with either growth hormone or zinc administration.

Key Question 3: Factors Associated With Treatment Efficacy

We found no consistent factors associated with better or poorer treatment outcome across studies. In medication studies, individuals with the nonbulimic subtype of AN had better therapeutic outcomes on cyprohoptadine than amitriptyline and placebo.[208] Bone density increased more in women with AN who were less than 70 percent of ideal body weight on estrogen replacement therapy.[210] These subgroup analyses had very small samples, and conclusions should be regarded as tentative.

One observation that was an artifact of experimental design,[223] post-weight restoration trial of CBT and nutritional counseling is related to patients being permitted to be on antidepressant medication. In one trial, a significantly higher percentage of CBT successes occurred among patients on medication. Miller et al.[211] reported that 3 weeks of transdermal testosterone was superior in decreasing depression in individuals who were depressed at baseline.

In terms of family therapy, Lock et al. found that adolescents with severe eating-related obsessive-compulsive-related thinking and those who come from nonintact families benefitted from longer-term rather than shorter-term manual-based family therapy treatment.[222] Eisler et al. found that families that scored higher on maternal criticism did better in separated rather than conjoint family therapy.[221]

Finally, with reference to weight gain, family therapy was more effective for AN patients whose illness began at an early age and had not become chronic.[231,239]

Key Question 4: Treatment Efficacy by Subgroups

The total number of individuals enrolled in the eight medication trials that reported the sex of the participants was 320. Of those, one was male. No medication studies reported differential outcome by age. With the exception of the one rGH trial[212] and one amitriptyline trial,[209] no medication studies have explicitly focused on the treatment of adolescent AN. Not a single medication study reported race or ethnicity of participants. Of the eight trials, seven were conducted in the United States and one in Canada. Based on these results, we conclude that no information exists regarding differential efficacy of pharmacotherapy interventions for AN by sex, gender, age, race, ethnicity, or cultural group.

The total number of individuals enrolled in the 11 psychotherapy trials was 572; of these, 22 were men or boys. Only two trials reported race or ethnicity of participants; they included eight Asian Americans, 10 Hispanic Americans, no African Americans, and three individuals of "other" race or ethnicity. In no instance were results analyzed specifically by race or ethnic group. No data exist regarding differential efficacy of psychotherapeutic treatment for AN by sex, gender, race, ethnicity, or cultural group.

In terms of age, scant evidence shows that interventions involving the family have greater efficacy for individuals below the age of 15 than for patients above that age. This information is based solely on studies by just one team of investigators who found family therapy to be more effective for adolescent AN patients with a shorter duration of illness than for adults with a more chronic course.[231,239] However, no definitive replications have been done. Moreover, no studies have explored the role of family therapy in adults focusing on the family of insertion rather than family of origin, which may be the relevant comparison, or other adaptation of family therapy for adults or adolescents.

Chapter 4. Results: Bulimia Nervosa

This chapter presents results of our literature search and our findings for the four key questions (KQs) that pertain to bulimia nervosa (BN), including the efficacy of various treatments or combinations of treatments (KQ 1), harms associated with the treatment or combination of treatments (KQ 2), factors associated with the efficacy of treatment (KQ 3), and whether the efficacy of treatment differs by sex, gender, age, race, ethnicity, or cultural groups (KQ 4).

We report specific details about the yields of the literature searches and characteristics of the studies. For each included study, detailed evidence tables appear in Appendix C.[**] We report first on medication trials (Evidence Table 5), then combined medication and behavioral interventions (Evidence Table 6), behavioral interventions (Evidence Table 7), self-help interventions (Evidence Table 8), and other interventions (Evidence Table 9). Within each evidence table, studies are listed alphabetically by author. Summary tables in this chapter present selected outcomes by type of intervention.

Overview of Included Studies

We identified 47 studies reported in 58 publications addressing treatment efficacy for BN. Of these, 14 were medication-only trials.[244-257] We rated two of these trials as good,[246,248] 9 as fair,[244,247,249-255,257] and three as poor.[245,256,258] The drugs studied included second-generation antidepressants,[244,247-250,252,254,255] tricyclic antidepressants,[257] an anticonvulsant,[251,259] monoamine-oxidase inhibitors (MAOIs),[253] and a 5HT3 antagonist.[246]

Six trials combined medication with behavioral interventions.[260-265] Three used second-generation antidepressants,[261,262,265] one used a tricyclic antidepressant,[260] and two used both a second-generation antidepressant and a tricyclic antidepressant sequentially.[263,264] Of these, we rated two as good[264,265] and four as fair.[260-263]

We identified 19 behavioral intervention psychotherapy studies published in 24 articles.[266-289] We rated three psychotherapy intervention trials as good,[269,270,282] 10 as fair,[266,273,274,276,278,280,281,283,287,288] and six as poor.[275,279,284-286,289] Of the 13 fair- and good-rated studies, 11 used some form of cognitive-behavioral therapy (CBT) in comparison to other interventions,[266,269,270,273,274,276,278,280,283,287,288] one used dialectical behavior therapy (DBT),[282] and one used nutritional management and stress management.[281]

We also identified five trials of various self-help methods.[290-294] We rated four as fair[290-293] and one as poor.[294]

Finally, we identified three studies of "other" interventions including active light,[295] guided imagery,[296] and crisis prevention.[297] We rated all three studies as fair.

Of the 47 studies addressing treatment efficacy for BN, we rated 10 as poor. Studies with a quality rating of "poor" are not discussed below. Reasons that these studies received this rating are presented in Table 12. Although each study was not lacking in all areas, the most common concerns contributing to the low rating included a fatal flaw in the approach to randomization or the approach not being described, assessors not being blinded or their blinding status not being described, adverse events not being reported, outcomes not being reported using an intention-to-

---

[**] Appendixes cited in this report are provided electronically at
http://www.ahrq.gov/downloads/pub/evidence/pdf/eatingdisorders/eatdis.pdf.

Table 12. Reasons for poor quality ratings and number of trials with poor ratings: bulimia nervosa

Reasons Contributing to Poor Ratings	Types of Intervention, Number of Times Flaw Was Detected, and Citations
Research Aims	
Hypothesis not clearly described	Medication-only trials: 0
	Behavioral intervention and self-help trials: 0
Study Population	
Characteristics not clearly described	Medication-only trials: 0
	Behavioral intervention and self-help trials: 1[289]
No specific inclusion or exclusion criteria	Medication-only trials: 0
	Behavioral intervention and self-help trials: 0
Randomization	
Protections against influence not in place	Medication-only trials: 0
	Behavioral intervention and self-help trials: 1[284]
Approach not described	Medication-only trials: 1[245]
	Behavioral intervention and self-help trials: 4[275,279,284,294,298]
Whether randomization had a fatal flaw not known	Medication-only trials: 2[245,256]
	Behavioral intervention and self-help trials: 6[275,279,284,286,289,294,298]
Comparison group(s) not similar at baseline	Medication-only trials: 2[245,256]
	Behavioral intervention and self-help trials: 1[289]
Blinding	
Study subjects	Medication-only trials: 0
	Behavioral intervention and self-help trials: 1[289]
Investigators	Medication-only trials: 0
	Behavioral intervention and self-help trials: 1[289]
Outcomes assessors	Medication-only trials: 2[245,256]
	Behavioral intervention and self-help trials: 7[275,279,284-286,289,294,298]
Interventions	
Interventions not clearly described	Medication-only trials: 0
	Behavioral intervention and self-help trials: 0
No reliable measurement of patient compliance	Medication-only trials: 1[256]
	Behavioral intervention and self-help trials: 3[279,285,289]
Outcomes	
Results not clearly described	Medication-only trials: 0
	Behavioral intervention and self-help trials: 0
Adverse events not reported	Medication-only trials: 0
	Behavioral intervention and self-help trials: 6[275,279,284-286,289]

Table 12. Reasons for poor quality ratings and number of trials with poor ratings: bulimia nervosa (continued)

Reasons Contributing to Poor Ratings	Types of Intervention, Number of Times Flaw Was Detected, and Citations
Statistical Analysis	
Statistics inappropriate	Medication-only trials: 0
	Behavioral intervention and self-help trials: 0
No controls for confounding (if needed)	Medication-only trials: 1[245]
	Behavioral intervention and self-help trials: 1[289]
Intention-to-treat analysis not used	Medication-only trials: 1[256]
	Behavioral intervention and self-help trials: 5[275,284-286,289]
Power analysis not done or not reported	Medication-only trials: 1[245]
	Behavioral intervention and self-help trials: 7[275,279,284-286,289,294,298]
Results	
Loss to followup 26% or higher or not reported	Medication-only trials: 0
	Behavioral intervention and self-help trials: 2[289,294,298]
Differential loss to followup 15% or higher or not reported	Medication-only trials: 1[245]
	Behavioral intervention and self-help trials: 3[275,286,289]
Outcome measures not standard, reliable, or valid in all groups	Medication-only trials: 0
	Behavioral intervention and self-help trials: 0
Discussion	
Results do not support conclusions, taking possible biases and limitations into account	Medication-only trials: 0
	Behavioral intervention and self-help trials: 0
Results not discussed within context of prior research	Medication-only trials: 1[256]
	Behavioral intervention and self-help trials: 0
External validity: population not representative of US population relevant to these treatments	Medication-only trials: 1[256]
	Behavioral intervention and self-help trials: 6[279,284-286,289,294,298]
Funding/sponsorship not reported	Medication-only trials: 0
	Behavioral intervention and self-help trials: 4[279,285,286,289]

treat approach, the statistical analysis not including a power analysis or not stating whether one was conducted, and concerns in relation to the external validity of the findings (the study population was not representative of the US population or the information of provided was insufficient to determine representativeness).

Participants

Of the 38 studies rated fair or good, 19 were conducted in the United States, five in Canada, four in Germany, three in the United Kingdom, two in Australia, and one each in Austria,

Finland, New Zealand, and Norway. In addition, one multinational trial had US and Canadian sites; another had German and Australian sites.

Of the fair and good studies, three failed to report the age of participants; of the remainder, the age range of participants was 16 to 61 years with the majority of participants being adults. A total of 3,403 individuals participated in fair or good clinical trials for BN. From those that reported sex, 2,985 women and 23 men participated.

Thirty-one studies failed to report the race or ethnicity of participants. Of those that did, 1,203 participants were identified as white, 79 as nonwhite, 27 as African American, 40 as Hispanic American, 30 as Asian or Pacific Islander, and one as Native American.

Similar to the AN studies, some BN trials also had high attrition. Table 13 documents the percentages of dropouts in total and in each arm of the study. Three studies had five study groups; those are combined with information relating to the fourth treatment group.

Key Question 1: Treatment Efficacy

Medication-only Trials

We report on 12 randomized controlled double-blind medication-only trials (Table 14). The total number of individuals enrolled was 1,430. Based on studies that reported sex, 1,364 women and 21 men participated in medication-only trials. The number of participants ranged from 26 to 398. The age of participants ranged from 16 to 55. Two trials reported the race of participants; in these, 521 individuals were reported as white and 27 as nonwhite. Seven trials were conducted in the United States, two in Canada, and one each in Australia, Germany, and Finland.

The medication-only trials used the following two designs: medication versus placebo (10) and medication (dose a) versus medication (dose b) versus placebo (1). The results of these studies are presented below by drug class.

Second-generation antidepressants. *Fluoxetine.* Six trials compared fluoxetine to placebo in outpatient and inpatient settings. The mean age of participants was mid-twenties; no studies of fluoxetine focused exclusively on adolescents.

Overall, fluoxetine (60 mg/day) administered for between 8 weeks and 16 weeks led to significant reductions in binge eating in most[244,249,250,254] but not all studies.[248,252] Fluoxetine (60 mg/day) also performed significantly better than fluoxetine (20 mg/day) in decreasing binge eating.[249] No effect of fluoxetine (60 mg/day) compared with placebo was observed in the one study in which patients were already receiving intensive inpatient psychotherapy.[248]

Fluoxetine (60 mg/day) was superior to placebo in decreasing purging behavior,[244,249,250,254] although not in the inpatient setting.[248]

All six fluoxetine trials either failed to report abstinence rates (absence of binge eating and purging behaviors) or did not report whether abstinence rates differed significantly between drug and placebo groups.

With reference to eating-related attitudes, fluoxetine (60 mg/day) was associated with significant improvements in measures of restraint, weight concern, and food preoccupation and with Eating Disorders Inventory (EDI) subscale scores of bulimia, drive for thinness, and body dissatisfaction.[244,249,250,254] Again, the exception was the inpatient study.[248]

Fluoxetine had mixed results on depression and anxiety scores. Some studies showed greater efficacy than placebo in decreasing depression scores,[249,252] but others showed no advantage of fluoxetine.[244,248,250,254]

Table 13. Dropout rates for randomized controlled trials: bulimia nervosa

Author	Total Enrollment, N	Total Dropouts N (% dropout)	G1 Treatment (% Dropout)	G2 Treatment (% Dropout)	G3 Treatment (% Dropout)	G4 Treatment (% Dropout) G5 Treatment (% Dropout)
		Medication Trial				
Beumont et al., 1997[244]	67	27 (40%)	Fluoxetine (50%)	Placebo (30%)		
Fichter et al., 1991[248]	39	0 (0%)	Fluoxetine (0%)	Placebo (0%)		
Fluoxetine BN Collaborative Study Group, 1992[249]	387	117 (30%)	Placebo (37%)	Fluoxetine, 20 mg (23%)	Fluoxetine, 60 mg (30%)	
Goldstein et al.,1995[250]	398	173 (43%)	Fluoxetine (40%)	Placebo (52%)		
Kanerva et al., 1995[252]	50	4 (8%)	Fluoxetine (8%)	Placebo (8%)		
Romano et al., 2002[254]	150	131 (87%)	Fluoxetine (83%)	Placebo (92%)		
Fichter et al., 1996[247] and Fichter et al., 1997[299]	72	24 (33%)	Fluvoxamine (51%)	Placebo (14%)		
Pope et al., 1989[255]	46	4 (9%)	Trazodone (13%)	Placebo (4%)		
Hoopes et al., 2003[251] and Hedges et al., 2003[259]	68	28 (41%)	Topiramate (34%)	Placebo (47%)		
Kennedy et al., 1993[253]	36	8 (21%)	Brofaromine (21%)	Placebo (24%)		
Faris et al., 2000[246]	26	1 (4%)	Ondansetron (7%)	Placebo (0%)		
Walsh et al., 1991[257]	78	15 (19%)	Placebo (16%)	Desipramine (23%)		
		Medication Plus Behavior Intervention Trials				
Goldbloom et al.,1997[261]	76	33 (43%)	Fluoxetine (39%)	CBT (35%)	Fluoxetine + CBT (55%)	
Mitchell et al., 2001[262]	91	2 (2%)	Placebo (5%)	Fluoxetine (0%)	Placebo + self-help manual (0%)	Fluoxetine + self-help manual (5%)
Walsh et al., 2004[265]	91	63 (69%)	Fluoxetine + guided self help (54%)	Placebo + guided self help (88%)	Fluoxetine (70%)	Placebo (64%)

B-ERP, exposure therapy with response prevention for bingeing; CBT, cognitive behavioral therapy; GP, general practitioner; IPT, interpersonal psychotherapy; N, number; NR, not reported; P-ERP, exposure therapy with response prevention for purging.

Table 13. Dropout rates for randomized controlled trials: bulimia nervosa (continued)

Author	Total Enrollment, N	Total Dropouts N (% dropout)	G1 Treatment (% Dropout)	G2 Treatment (% Dropout)	G3 Treatment (% Dropout)	G4 Treatment (% Dropout) G5 Treatment (% Dropout)
Agras et al., 1992[260] and Agras et al., 1994[300]	71	18 (25%)	Desipramine 16 weeks (NR)	Desipramine 24 weeks (NR)	Desipramine 16 weeks + CBT (NR)	Desipramine 24 weeks + CBT (NR) CBT (NR)
Mitchell et al., 2002[263]	62	25 (40%)	IPT (32%)	Antidepressant medication (48%)		
Walsh et al., 1997[264] and Wilson et al., 1999[301]	120	41 (34%)	CBT + medication (NR)	CBT + Placebo (NR)	Supportive therapy + medication (NR)	Supportive therapy + placebo (NR) Medication only (43%)
Behavioral Intervention Trials						
Agras et al., 2000[269]	220	57 (26%)	CBT (28%)	IPT (24%)		
Wolk and Devlin, 2001[268]	110	44 (40%)	CBT (NR)	IPT (NR)		
Cooper and Steere, 1995[274]	31	4 (13%)	CBT (13%)	Behavioral therapy (13%)		
Fairburn et al., 1991[276] and Fairburn et al., 1993[267]	75	15 (20%)	CBT (16%)	Behavioral therapy (24%)	IPT (12%)	
Wilfley et al., 1993[287]	56	8 (14%)	CBT (33%)	IPT (11%)	Waiting list (0%)	
Wilson et al., 2002[288]	220	Post treatment: 66 (30%), Follow up: 91 (41%)	CBT (NR)	IPT (NR)		
Garner et al., 1993[278]	60	10 (17%)	CBT (17%)	Supportive expressive (17%)		
Hsu et al., 2001[280]	100	27 (27%)	Nutritional therapy (39%)	Cognitive therapy (15%)	Cognitive and nutritional therapy (11%)	Sequential group (46%)
Sundgot-Borgen et al., 2002[283]	64	6 (9%)	Exercise (20%)	CBT (13%)	Nutrition (0%)	Waiting list (6%) Healthy control (0%)
Chen et al., 2003[273]	60	16 (27%)	Individual CBT (27%)	Group CBT (27%)		
Agras et al., 1989[266]	77	67 (13%)	Waiting list (5%)	Self monitoring (16%)	CBT (23%)	CBT + response prevention (6%)

Table 13. Dropout rates for randomized controlled trials: bulimia nervosa (continued)

Author	Total Enrollment	Total Dropouts N (% dropout)	G1 Treatment (% Dropout)	G2 Treatment (% Dropout)	G3 treatment (% Dropout)	G4 Treatment (% Dropout) G5 Treatment (% Dropout)
Bulik et al., 1998[270] and Bulik et al.,1998[271]	111	5 (5%)	Exposure to B-ERP (5%)	Exposure to P-ERP (6%)	Relaxation training (3%)	
Laessle et al., 1991[281]	55	7 (13%)	Nutritional management (19%)	Stress management (7%)		
Safer, Telch, and Agras, 2001[282]	31	2 (6%)	Dialectical behavior therapy (13%)	Waiting list (7%)		
Self-help Trials						
Bailer et al., 2004[290]	81	25 (31%)	Self help (25%)	CBT (37%)		
Carter et al., 2003[291]	85	20 (24%)	CBT (18%)	Nonspecific (25%)	Waiting list (28%)	
Durand and King, 2003[292]	68	14 (21%)	GP self-help (24%)	Specialist treatment (18%)		
Thiels et al., 1998[293]	62	13 (21%)	CBT (13%)	Guided self change (29%)		
Other Interventions						
Braun et al., 1999[295]	34	10 (29%)	Active light (31%)	Dim light (28%)		
Mitchell et al., 2004[297]	57	17 weeks: 9 (16%); 43 weeks: 16 (28%), 70 weeks: 23 (40%)	Crisis prevention 17 weeks: (10%), 43 weeks: (23%), 70 weeks: (37%)	Follow up 17 weeks: (22%), 43 weeks: (33%), 70 weeks: (44%)		
Esplen et al., 1998[296]	58	8 (14%)	Guided imagery (14%)	Control (13%)		

Table 14. Results from medication trials: bulimia nervosa

Source, Treatment, Setting, and Quality Score	Major Outcome Measures	Significant Change Over Time Within Groups	Significant Differences Between Groups at Endpoint	Significant Differences Between Groups in Change Over Time
Beumont, Russell et al., 1997[244] Fluoxetine vs. placebo Outpatient Fair	Eating: • BSQ • Bulimic episodes • EAT • EDE • Vomiting Biomarker: • Weight Psych: • HDRS	Both groups decreased bulimic and vomiting episodes, ED concerns and symptoms; and worries about body shape at week 4. Both groups decreased bulimic and vomiting episodes; ED concerns and symptoms; worries about body shape; restraint, overeating, and concerns about eating, shape, and weight at week 8. Both groups decreased bulimic and vomiting episodes, restraint, overeating, and concerns about eating and shape at 3-month FU. Fluoxetine group increased weight at 3 month FU.	Fluoxetine associated with lower restraint, weight concern, and shape concern at week 8	Significant difference on weight at 8 weeks with weight decreasing in fluoxetine group and increasing in placebo group. Fluoxetine group regained weight above baseline at FU while placebo group did not.
Fichter et al., 1991[248] Fluoxetine vs. placebo Inpatient Good	Eating: • Binge attacks • Binge urge • EDI • SIAB Biomarker: • Weight Psych: • CGI • HAM-D • SCL-90	No statistics reported.	No differences on any measures.	No differences on any measures.

BDI, Beck Depression Inventory; BITE, Bulimic Investigation Test Edinburgh; BMI, Body mass index; BSQ, Body Shape Questionnaire; CGI, Clinical Global Impression Scale; EAT, Eating Attitudes Test [EAT-26 items]; ED, Eating disorder; EDE, Eating Disorder Examination; EDI, Eating Disorders Inventory; FU, followup; HAM-A, Hamilton Anxiety Index; HAM-D (or HDRS), Hamilton Depression Rating Scale [HDRS-17 items, HDRS-21 items]; HRSD, Hamilton Rating Depression Scale; HSCL, Hopkins Symptom Check List (see SCL-90); kg, kilogram; PGI, Patient Global Impression; Psych, psychiatric and psychological; SCL, (Hopkins) Symptom Check List (SCL-90 items); SIAB, Structured Interview for Anorexia and Bulimia nervosa; STAI, Spielberger State-Trait Anxiety Inventory; tx, treatment; YBC-EDS, Yale-Brown-Cornell Eating Disorder Scale.

Table 14. Results from medication trials: bulimia nervosa (continued)

Source, Treatment, Setting, and Quality Score	Major Outcome Measures	Significant Change Over Time Within Groups	Significant Differences Between Groups at Endpoint	Significant Differences Between Groups in Change Over Time
Fluoxetine BN Collaborative Study Group, 1992[249] Fluoxetine (20 mg) vs. fluoxetine (60 mg) vs. placebo Outpatient Fair	Eating: • Bingeing • Vomiting • EAT • EDI • Carbohydrate craving Biomarker: • Weight Psych: • HDRS	No statistics reported.	Fluoxetine (60 mg) associated with greater reductions in binge eating and vomiting than fluoxetine (20 mg) or placebo. Fluoxetine (60 mg and 20 mg) associated with greater reductions in vomiting, weight, drive for thinness, bulimic intensity, carbohydrate craving, body dissatisfaction, and food and diet preoccupation than placebo. Fluoxetine (60 mg) associated with greater reductions in depressed mood, drive for thinness, oral control, and bulimia scores than placebo.	No statistics reported.
Goldstein, Wilson, Thompson et al., 1995[250] Fluoxetine vs. placebo Outpatient Fair	Eating: • Binge eating • Vomiting • EDI Biomarker: • Weight Psych: • CGI • HRSD • PGI	No statistics reported.	Fluoxetine associated with greater median percentage reduction in vomiting (at weeks 1-10, 13, 16, and endpoint) and binge eating (at weeks 1-9, 13, 16, and endpoint); greater reduction in total bulimia symptoms, drive for thinness, global symptoms scores, and weight; greater tx response (≥ 50% improvement in bulimic episodes)	No statistics reported.
Kanerva, Rissanen, and Sarna, 1994[252] Fluoxetine vs. placebo Outpatient Fair	Eating: • Bingeing • BITE • EAT • EDI Biomarker: • Weight Psych: • HDRS-17 • HDRS-21 • STAI	At 4 weeks, fluoxetine group decreased anxious mood and state anxiety.	No statistics reported.	Fluoxetine associated with greater reduction in depressed and anxious mood, bulimia and food preoccupation over 8 weeks. Difference in weight with decrease in fluoxetine group and increase in placebo group.

65

Table 14. Results from medication trials: bulimia nervosa (continued)

Source, Treatment, Setting, and Quality Score	Major Outcome Measures	Significant Change Over Time Within Groups	Significant Differences Between Groups at Endpoint	Significant Differences Between Groups in Change Over Time
Romano et al., 2002[254] Fluoxetine vs. placebo Outpatient Fair	Eating: • Bingeing • EDI • Relapse • Vomiting • YBC-EDS Biomarker: • BMI Psych: • CGI • HDRS	Both groups worsened over the 52-week extended tx period.	No statistics reported.	Fluoxetine group had smaller mean increases in vomiting, binge eating, total ED behavior, ritual, preoccupation and symptom severity. Relapse occurred less frequently in the first 3 months of 52-week extended tx period.
Fichter et al., 1996[247] Fichter et al., 1997[299] Fluvoxamine vs. placebo Inpatient and outpatient Fair	Eating: • Abstinence • Bingeing • EDI • Relapse • SIAB • Urge to binge Biomarker: • BMI Psych: • CGI • HDRS • HSCL	No statistics reported.	Fluvoxamine associated with higher binge abstinence rate, reduced clinical severity, and lower relapse rate.	Fluvoxamine superior in limiting increases in bulimic behavior (urge to binge, vomiting), global ED symptoms (SIAB total), EDI bulimia scores, fear of losing control, obsessive-compulsive symptoms, and, global severity during 12 week post-discharge relapse prevention phase.
Pope et al., 1989[255] Trazadone vs. placebo Outpatient Fair	Eating: • Binge frequency • EDI • Vomit frequency • Fear of eating Psych: • Self-control • Self-esteem • HAM-A • HAM-D	Trazadone group decreased binge and purge frequencies and fear of eating at 6 wks.	Trazadone associated greater percent decrease in binge and vomit frequencies and decrease in fear of eating and increase in self-esteem.	No statistics reported.

Table 14. Results from medication trials: bulimia nervosa (continued)

Source, Treatment, Setting, and Quality Score	Major Outcome Measures	Significant Change Over Time Within Groups	Significant Differences Between Groups at Endpoint	Significant Differences Between Groups in Change Over Time
Hoopes et al., 2003;[251] Hedges et al., 2003[259] Topiramate vs. placebo Outpatient Fair	Eating: • Binge days • Bulimic intensity scale • Carbohydrate craving • EAT • EDI • Purge days • Remission Biomarker: • Weight Psych: • CGI • HAM-A • HAM-D • PGI	No statistics reported.	Topiramate associated with greater percentage reduction in weekly number of binge and purge days, carbohydrate craving score, bulimic intensity, lower mean global symptoms and symptom intensity; and greater mean weight reduction. Larger percentage of topiramate group achieved moderate (> 50% reduction) or marked (> 75% reduction) improvement in weekly binge/purge days.	Topiramate superior to placebo in reducing uncontrolled eating, body dissatisfaction, dieting, food preoccupation, and anxious mood, and in increasing patient-rated percent improved.
Kennedy et al., 1993[253] Brofaromine vs. placebo Outpatient Fair	Eating: • Binge episodes • EAT-26 • EDI • Non-binge meals • Vomiting episodes Biomarker: • BMI • Weight Psych: • HAM-A • HAM-D	No statistics reported.	Brofaromine associated with greater reduction in vomiting episodes. A greater percentage of brofaromine group lost > 1 kg of weight. A greater percentage of placebo group gained > 1 kg of weight.	No statistics reported
Faris et al., 2000[246] Ondansetron vs. placebo Inpatient and outpatient Good	Eating: • Binge-purge episodes • Normal meals • Time spent in BN behaviors Biomarker: • Weight	Ondansetron group increased average number of normal meals, and decreased time spent engaging in BN behaviors at week 4.	Ondansetron associated with lower binge/purge frequency at week 4.	Ondansetron superior in reducing binge/vomit frequency and time spent engaging in BN behaviors and in increasing normal meals over 4 weeks.

Table 14. Results from medication trials: bulimia nervosa (continued)

Source, Treatment, Setting, and Quality Score	Major Outcome Measures	Significant Change Over Time Within Groups	Significant Differences Between Groups at Endpoint	Significant Differences Between Groups in Change Over Time
Walsh et al., 1991[257] Desipramine vs. placebo Outpatient Fair	Eating: • Binge episodes • BSQ • EAT • Remission • Vomiting episodes Biomarker: • BMI Psych: • BDI • HAM-D • SCL-90 • Social adjustment scale • STAI	No statistics reported.	Desipramine associated with fewer binge and vomiting episodes/week, fewer ED symptoms and body shape concerns, lower BMI, fewer symptoms of depression, global symptoms, and obsessive/compulsiveness, less hostility and trait anxiety.	No statistics reported.

One study explored the efficacy of fluoxetine (60 mg/day) versus placebo in preventing relapse of BN over 52 weeks.[254] Relapse rates were significantly lower for those receiving fluoxetine (33 percent) than for those receiving placebo (51 percent). However, dropout was substantial during the observation period (83 percent in the fluoxetine group and 92 percent in the placebo group).

Drop-out rates in fluoxetine arms of these trials ranged from zero (in an inpatient study) to 50 percent (three studies had greater than 40 percent dropout). In one study, dropout was greater in the fluoxetine than in the placebo group,[244] in three studies placebo had greater attrition,[249,250,254] and one inpatient study reported no dropout in either group.[248]

Fluvoxamine. To compare maintenance of therapeutic gains and prevention of relapse of BN after inpatient treatment, Fichter et al. compared fluvoxamine (average dose 182 mg/day) with placebo for 19 weeks.[247] Patients treated with fluvoxamine reported fewer urges to binge, lower frequency of vomiting, and lower depression scores than those receiving placebo. Both groups gained weight, with no differences between groups. Fluvoxamine was associated with a lower relapse rate. However, attrition was high (51 percent for those on fluvoxamine and 14 percent for those on placebo).

Trazodone. In a 6-week trial of trazodone (400 mg) versus placebo, trazodone led to significantly greater decreases in the frequency of binge eating and vomiting and decreased fear of eating.[255] No differences in depression or anxiety were observed, although baseline levels were not indicative of severe depression.

Tricyclic antidepressants. One 6-week trial of desipramine (200-300 mg/day) versus placebo found the active drug to be significantly more effective than placebo in decreasing binge eating, vomiting, and scores on the Eating Attitudes Test (EAT) and Body Shape Questionnaire (BSQ).[257] Abstinence rates from binge eating and purging did not differ between active drug and placebo. Both self-reported depression and anxiety were significantly decreased in the desipramine group compared with the placebo group; clinician-rated depression did not differ significantly. Patients in the desipramine group lost significantly more weight than those in the placebo group, who tended to gain weight. Dropout was 23 percent in the desipramine group and 16 percent in the placebo group.

Anticonvulsants. The single 10-week trial of the anticonvulsant topiramate (mean dose 100 mg/day) led to significantly greater reductions than placebo in the number of binge/purge days reported and in body dissatisfaction, drive for thinness, and EAT scores.[251,259] Abstinence rates from binge eating and purging were 22.6 percent for topiramate and 6 percent for placebo (not significantly different). Topiramate was associated with significant reductions in anxiety but not depression, and the topiramate group lost significantly more weight than the placebo group, who tended to gain weight. Dropout from topiramate treatment was 34 percent and 47 percent for placebo.

MAOI. One 8-week trial of brofaromine (mean dose 175 mg/day) revealed no differences between the active drug and placebo on binge eating or psychological features of the eating disorder.[253] Brofaromine did lead to significant reductions in vomiting. Abstinence from binge eating and from vomiting were measured independently and did not differ between groups; no differences were observed on depression or anxiety scores, weight change, or drop-out rates (21 percent brofaromine and 24 percent placebo).

5HT3 antagonist. In a small 4-week trial of ondansetron versus placebo—self-administered when patients had an urge to binge or vomit—the active drug led to significantly greater decreases than placebo in binge and vomit frequencies and time spent in bulimic behavior, and to significant increases in normal meals.[246] The investigators did not measure depression or anxiety, and they found no differences in weight change. One patient dropped out from ondansetron, none from placebo.

Summary of medication-only trials. Fluoxetine (60 mg/day) administered for 6 to 18 weeks has been shown in several fair- to good-rated trials to reduce the core bulimia symptoms of binge eating and purging and associated psychological features of the eating disorder in the short term. The 60 mg dose performs better than the 20 mg dose;[249] it was also associated with prevention of relapse at 1 year in a study with considerable dropout.[254] Considerable evidence exists for the use of 60 mg/day of fluoxetine to treat BN in the short term. Evidence for the long-term effectiveness of relatively brief medication treatment does not exist. The optimal duration of treatment and the optimal strategy for maintenance of treatment gains are unknown.

Single studies provide preliminary evidence of the efficacy of two other second-generation antidepressants, namely trazodone[255] and fluvoxamine.[247] Likewise, evidence from single studies provides preliminary evidence of the efficacy of desipramine[257] and topiramate.[251] One preliminary trial of ondansetron, a 5HT3 antagonist and antiemetic, led to an intriguing decrease in binge eating and vomiting when patients could self-administer when they had urges to binge or purge.[246] This innovative study requires replication. One trial of brofaromine, an MAOI, showed a significantly greater effect on reducing vomiting than placebo.[253]

When reported, abstinence rates in medication-only trials suggest that medication treatment leads to abstinence in a minority of individuals. This finding indicates that although bulimia symptoms improved, they nonetheless persisted.

Drop-out rates in medication trials ranged from zero to 51 percent. No drug showed substantially greater attrition than others.

Medication Plus Behavioral Intervention Trials

We present the six trials of medications plus behavioral interventions in Table 15. These trials used a variety of designs to determine the extent to which a combination intervention is superior to either medication or behavioral intervention alone.

The total number of individuals enrolled in these combination trials was 1,895. The number of participants in the medication plus psychotherapy trials ranged from 71 to 120. No men participated in these trials. Participant ages ranged from 18 to 46. Three trials reported race or ethnicity of participants: 272 individuals were reported to be white, seven nonwhite, two Hispanic American, eight African American, and seven Asian. Five of these trials were conducted in the United States and one in Canada.

Second-generation antidepressants and CBT. Three trials used fluoxetine as the drug intervention. Comparing fluoxetine (60 mg/day) to CBT only to fluoxetine (60 mg/day) plus CBT in a 12-week trial, Goldbloom et al. used intention-to-treat analyses but found no difference across groups on eating related-measures.[261] In completers, all three interventions led to significant improvement in core bulimic symptoms; however, both combined treatment and CBT alone led to greater decreases than fluoxetine alone in objective and subjective binges and vomiting episodes. Abstinence rates, depression scores, and weight did not differ across groups. Dropout was highest in combined treatment (55 percent) compared to the fluoxetine (39 percent) and CBT only groups (35 percent). The investigators did not provide long-term followup data.

Walsh et al. compared fluoxetine (60 mg/day) with placebo, each with or without self-help in the form of a cognitive-behavioral self-help book[302] with instructions for use.[265] Physicians and nurses in primary care provided the treatments. Fluoxetine (either alone or with self-help) was associated with significantly decreased objective binge episodes, vomiting, restrained eating, and depression. The self-help book had no independent effect. No differences emerged on weight change. Dropout was high: 54 percent in fluoxetine plus guided self-help to 88 percent in placebo plus guided self-help.

Using the same design but a different self-help manual, also based on principles of CBT, and administering treatment from a specialized eating disorders program, Mitchell et al. found fluoxetine to be associated with a significantly greater decrease than placebo in vomiting episodes but not binge eating episodes.[262] No significant differences emerged in abstinence rates or depression. At the end of treatment, the investigators reported no independent effect of self-help. Dropout was low: none in fluoxetine only and fluoxetine plus self-help, 5 percent in placebo only and placebo plus self-help.

Tricyclic antidepressants and CBT. One complex trial compared desipramine treatment of different durations with or without CBT (16 versus 24 weeks) with CBT only.[260] The 16-week combined treatment was better than drug only for decreasing binge eating and purging. Longer combined treatment was significantly better than drug only on binge eating, vomiting, dieting preoccupation, and hunger. Abstinence rates did not differ across groups. The authors did not report results concerning depression. Weight change did not differ significantly across groups. At 1-year followup, the combined 24-week intervention and CBT alone were both better than the 16-week drug only treatment in decreasing binge eating and vomiting. The 24-week combined treatment was also superior to 16-week drug only in decreasing binge frequency, dietary preoccupation, disinhibition, and hunger.[300] In all but the medication-only group, between 78 percent and 100 percent of individuals who were abstinent at the end of treatment remained abstinent at followup. The overall drop-out rate was 25 percent.

Table 15. Results from medication plus behavioral intervention trials: bulimia nervosa

Source, Treatment, Setting, and Quality Score	Major Outcome Measures	Significant Change Over Time Within Groups	Significant Differences Between Groups at Endpoint	Significant Differences Between Groups in Change Over Time
Goldbloom et al., 1997[261] Fluoxetine vs. CBT vs. fluoxetine + CBT Outpatient Fair	Eating: • Binge episodes • EDE • EDI • Vomiting episodes Biomarker: • Weight Psych: • BDI • RSE	Decreased shape and weight concerns in the fluoxetine and the fluoxetine + CBT groups.	At tx completion, CBT alone and fluoxetine + CBT associated with greater percent reduction in vomiting frequency, compared to fluoxetine alone. At 4 weeks post-tx, fluoxetine + CBT associated with fewer objective binge and vomit weekly episodes compared to fluoxetine alone. CBT associated with fewer subjective binge episodes compared to fluoxetine alone. Note: no sig diff in ITT analyses.	No statistics reported.
Mitchell et al., 2001[262] Fluoxetine vs. placebo vs. self-help + placebo vs. fluoxetine + self-help Outpatient Fair	Eating: • Abstinence • Binge eating • EDI • Fasting days • Vomiting Psych: • CGI • HAM-D • PGI	No statistics reported.	Fluoxetine, alone and with self-help, associated with greater percentage reduction in vomiting and greater clinician-rated and patient-rated clinical improvement, compared to self help plus placebo or placebo alone, at endpoint (16 week tx period). Self-help manual plus placebo or fluoxetine associated with greater percentage reduction in vomiting compared to placebo or fluoxetine with no self-help manual, at 4-week time point (after 2 weeks active tx).	No statistics reported.

BDI, Beck Depression Inventory; BES, Binge Eating Scale; BMI, body mass index; BSQ, Body Shape Questionnaire; CBT, cognitive behavior therapy; CGI, clinical global impression; EAT, Eating Attitudes Test; ED, eating disorders; EDE, eating disorders examination; EDI, eating disorder inventory; FU, followup; HAM-D, Hamilton Rating Score for Depression; ITT, intention-to-treat; IPT, interpersonal psychotherapy; PGI, patient global impression; Psych, psychiatric and psychological; RSE, Rosenberg Self-Esteem Questionnaire; SCL, (Hopkins) Symptom Checklist (SCL-53 items, SCL-90 items); TFEQ, Three Factor Eating Questionnaire; tx, treatment; vs., versus; YBC-ED, Yale-Brown-Cornell Eating Disorder Scale.

Table 15. Results from medication plus behavioral intervention trials: bulimia nervosa (continued)

Source, Treatment, Setting, and Quality Score	Major Outcome Measures	Significant Change Over Time Within Groups	Significant Differences Between Groups at Endpoint	Significant Differences Between Groups in Change Over Time
Walsh et al., 2004[265] Fluoxetine vs. placebo vs. guided self-help vs. fluoxetine + guided self-help Outpatient Good	Eating: • EDE (episodes of bulimia, laxative use, vomiting) • Restraint Biomarker: • BMI Psych: • BDI • SCL-53	No statistics reported.	Fluoxetine associated with fewer objective bulimic and vomiting episodes and fewer vomiting days per month, less restraint, less depressed mood, and a lower general symptom index compared to placebo. Fluoxetine only and placebo groups greater decrease in bulimic episodes than self-help groups.	No statistics reported
Agras et al., 1992;[260] and Agras et al., 1994[300] Desipramine (16 weeks) vs. desipramine (24 weeks) vs. desipramine + CBT (16 weeks) vs. desipramine + CBT (24 weeks) vs. CBT alone (24 weeks) Outpatient Fair	Eating: • Abstinence • Bingeing • Dietary pre-occupation • Disinhibition • EDE • Hunger • Purging • Recovery Biomarker: • Weight Psych: • BDI • RSE	No statistics reported.	No statistics reported.	Desipramine + CBT superior to medication alone in reducing binge and purge frequency at 16 and 32 weeks, and in reducing diet preoccupation over 16 weeks. Desipramine + CBT superior to CBT alone in reducing hunger disinhibition over 24 weeks, and superior to medication alone in reducing diet preoccupation at 16 weeks. CBT alone superior to desipramine alone for 16 or 24 wks in reducing binge and purge frequency at 16 wks. CBT alone or in combination with desipramine for 24 weeks, superior to desipramine for 16 weeks in reducing binge frequency at 1 year FU. Desipramine + CBT for 24 weeks superior to desipramine for 16 weeks in reducing binge frequency, hunger, disinhibition, and diet preoccupation at 1 year FU.

Table 15. Results from medication plus behavioral intervention trials: bulimia nervosa (continued)

Source, Treatment, Setting, and Quality Score	Major Outcome Measures	Significant Change Over Time Within Groups	Significant Differences Between Groups at Endpoint	Significant Differences Between Groups in Change Over Time
Mitchell et al., 2002[263] IPT vs. fluoxetine (16 weeks) or vs. fluoxetine (8 weeks) followed by desipramine (8 weeks) Outpatient Fair	Eating: • Abstinence • BES • BSQ • EDE • Objective binges • Relapse • TFEQ Psych: • BDI	No statistics reported.	No differences on any measures.	No statistics reported.
Walsh et al., 1997[264] and Wilson et al., 1999[301] CBT + placebo vs. CBT + medication (desipramine only or desipramine followed by fluoxetine) vs. Supportive therapy + placebo vs. Supportive therapy + medication vs. Medication alone Outpatient Good	Eating: • Bingeing • BSQ • EAT • EDE • Remittance • Vomiting Biomarker: • BMI • Weight Psych: • BDI • SCL-90	All groups exhibited decreases in weekly bingeing and vomiting, EAT and BSQ scores, concerns about eating and eating restraint, global ED symptoms, and depressed mood. Weight and BMI decreased in 3 groups (CBT+ placebo, medication alone, and supportive therapy + medication). Anxiety decreased in each of the 3 groups receiving medication. Importance of shape and weight concerns decreased in two groups (CBT plus placebo and supportive therapy plus medication).	No statistics reported.	CBT groups combined superior to supportive therapy groups combined in reducing binge and vomit episode frequencies. Behavioral interventions plus medication superior to behavioral interventions alone in reducing binge frequency, EAT scores, depressed mood, weight, and in increasing remission rate. CBT plus medication superior to medication alone in reducing binge and vomit frequencies, EAT scores, body image, and increasing remission rate by self-report. Medication alone superior to CBT alone in reducing BMI and weight. Medication alone superior to supportive therapy plus medication in reducing binge and vomit frequency.

Multiple drugs and CBT. Walsh et al. examined supportive psychotherapy, CBT, both with or without placebo and with or without medication, and medication alone in a five-group 16-week comparison.[264,301] They started patients on desipramine (mean dose 188 mg/day) and switched nonresponders to fluoxetine (60 mg/day) after 8 weeks. Analyses combining all arms of the study that included CBT versus all arms of the study that included supportive therapy indicated that CBT was superior to supportive therapy in reducing binge and vomit episode frequencies. Behavioral interventions plus medication were superior to behavioral interventions alone in reducing binge frequency, EAT scores, depressed mood, weight, and in increasing remission rate.

CBT plus medication was superior to medication alone in reducing binge and vomit frequencies, EAT scores, body image, and increasing remission rate by self-report. Medication alone was superior to CBT alone in reducing BMI and weight. Medication alone was superior to supportive therapy plus medication in reducing binge and vomit frequency. Medication led to significantly greater decreases in depression scores. CBT was associated with greater likelihood of remission. The overall drop-out rate was 34 percent.

Mitchell et al. randomized patients who did not respond to CBT to either interpersonal psychotherapy or fluoxetine (60 mg/day), which could be switched to desipramine in those who did not achieve abstinence.[263] No difference in abstinence was observed between the two groups. Overall, the sequential second-level treatment was associated with high dropout.

Summary of medication plus psychotherapy trials. The combined medication plus behavioral intervention studies provide only preliminary evidence regarding the optimal combination of medication and psychotherapy or self-help. Given the variety of designs used and lack of replication, evidence remains weak. Combined CBT and fluoxetine and CBT alone led to greater decreases in binge eating and purging than fluoxetine alone in individuals who complete therapy.[261] When delivered in the context of a specialist eating disorders program, both self-help and fluoxetine were associated with decreased vomiting; however, the addition of self-help to fluoxetine was not associated with increased efficacy.[262] When these therapies were administered in a primary care setting, drop-out rates from fluoxetine (70 percent) and fluoxetine plus self-help (54 percent) were unacceptably high.[265]

The only study that looked at sequential treatment for individuals who did not respond to CBT revealed that the addition of interpersonal psychotherapy to fluoxetine (allowing the transition to desipramine) led to substantial attrition and minimal effects on subsequent abstinence rates. How best to treat individuals who do not respond to CBT or fluoxetine remains a major shortcoming of the literature.

Behavioral Intervention Trials

We report 13 psychotherapy-only trials, four self-help trials, one trial of light therapy, one of guided imagery, and one of crisis prevention. Summary outcomes data for the psychotherapy trials appear in Table 16. The total number of individuals enrolled in psychotherapy, self-help, and other trials was 1,462. From the studies that reported sex of participants, 1,064 women and two men participated. Across these 20 trials, participants ranged in age from 17 to 64 years. Six trials reported race and ethnicity of participants: in all, 410 patients were white; 22 nonwhite; 28 Hispanic American; 26 Asian, Maori, or Pacific Islander; 10 African American; and 1 Native American. In no instance were results analyzed specifically by race or ethnicity group. Of the 20 trials, seven were conducted in the United States, three each in Canada and the United Kingdom, one each in Australia, Austria, Germany, New Zealand, and Norway, and one two-site study in Germany and Australia, and one did not report location.

Psychotherapy trials for bulimia nervosa. *Cognitive Behavior Therapy.* CBT focusing on cognitive and behavioral factors that maintain bulimic behaviors is the most widely studied intervention for BN. Eleven trials of various designs delivered CBT either individually or in group format. CBT was compared with interpersonal psychotherapy (IPT),[269,276,287,288] with supportive expressive therapy,[278] with nutritional counseling,[280,283] and with exercise.[283] One study compared individually with group-administered CBT.[273] Several studies dismantled CBT by comparing complete CBT with behavioral therapy (BT) in the absence of a cognitive component,[276] by comparing cognitive therapy only with exposure with response prevention

Table 16. Results from behavioral intervention trials: bulimia nervosa

Source, Treatment, Setting, and Quality Score	Major Outcome Measures	Significant Change Over Time Within Groups	Significant Differences Between Groups at Endpoint	Significant Differences Between Groups in Change Over Time
Agras et al., 2000[269] and Wolk and Devlin, 2001[268] CBT vs. IPT Outpatient Good	Eating: • Bingeing • EDE • Purging • Remittance • Recovery Biomarker: • BMI Psych: • SCL-90R • Stage of change	No statistics reported.	CBT associated with higher percent remitted and percent recovered at end of tx (ITT analysis). In completers-only analysis, CBT associated with fewer objective binges and purges; less eating restraint; and less weight, shape, and eating concerns at the end of tx. Stage of change predicted improvement in IPT but not CBT.	No statistics reported.
Cooper and Steere, 1995[274] Cognitive therapy vs. exposure plus binge and purge response prevention Outpatient Fair	Eating: • Abstinence • Bulimic episodes • BSQ • EAT • EDE • Dietary restraint • Relapse • Vomiting episodes Biomarker: • Weight Psych: • BDI • PSE • MADRS • STAI	No statistics reported.	Relapse rate lower in cognitive therapy group among those who were abstinent from binge-eating at end of tx and at 12 month FU.	Cognitive therapy superior to exposure therapy in reducing vomiting and depression between baseline and 12 month FU.

B-ERP, exposure with response prevention to pre-binge cues; BDI, Beck Depression Inventory; BMI, Body mass index; BN, bulimia nervosa; BSQ, Body Shape Questionnaire; BT, Behavioral Therapy; CBT, Cognitive Behavioral Therapy; CNT, Cognitive nutritional therapy; CT, Cognitive Therapy; DBT, dialectical behavior therapy; EAT, Eating Attitudes Test; ED, Eating disorder; EDE, Eating Disorder Examination (EDE-12 items); EDI, Eating Disorders Inventory; FU, follow-up; GAFS, Global Assessment of Functioning Symptoms; HDRS, Hamilton Depression Rating Scale; IIP, Inventory of Interpersonal Problems; IPT, interpersonal psychotherapy; ITT, intention-to-treat; MADRS, Montgomery and Asberg Depression Rating Scale; NT, nutritional therapy; P-ERP, exposure with response prevention to pre-purge cues; PSE, Present State Examination; Psych, psychiatric and psychological; RSE, Rosenberg Self-Esteem Scale; SCL-90, (Hopkins) symptom checklist (SCL-90 items, SFL-90-R [SCL-90-revised]); STAI, Speilberger State-Trait Anxiety Inventory; SUDS, subjective units of distress; TFEQ, Three Factor Eating Questionnaire; tx, treatment.

Table 16. Results from behavioral intervention trials: bulimia nervosa (continued)

Source, Treatment, Setting, and Quality Score	Major Outcome Measures	Significant Change Over Time Within Groups	Significant Differences Between Groups at Endpoint	Significant Differences Between Groups in Change Over Time
Fairburn et al., 1991;[276] Fairburn, Jones et al., 1993[267] and Fairburn, Peveler et al., 1993[277] CBT vs. BT vs. IPT Outpatient Fair	Eating: • EAT • EDE • Laxative misuse • Objective bulimic episodes • Vomiting Biomarker: • BMI Psych: • BDI • SCL-90 • RSE	No statistics reported.	No statistics reported.	Over 18 week tx period, CBT superior to BT and IPT in reducing eating restraint, weight concerns, and overall ED psychopathology; CBT superior to IPT in reducing vomiting; and CBT superior to BT in reducing shape concerns. Over 12-month FU, CBT superior to BT in improving abstinence.
Wilfley et al., 1993[287] Group CBT vs. group IPT vs. waiting-list control Outpatient Fair	Eating: • Binge frequency • EDE • TFEQ Psych: • BDI • IIP • RSE	CBT and IPT decreased binge frequency at 1 year FU.	No statistics reported.	Group CBT and group IPT superior to waiting-list in reducing binge frequency, and disinhibition over 16 weeks. Group IPT superior to waiting-list in reducing restraint over 16 weeks.
Wilson et al., 2002[288] CBT vs. IPT Outpatient Fair	Eating: • Binge eating • EDE • Recovery • Vomiting Psych: • IIP • RSE • Self-efficacy	Both groups decreased shape and weight concerns at post-tx.	CBT showed greater mean reduction in eating restraint by tx week 6, greater improvements in self-efficacy by tx week 10, and a higher percentage reduction in binge eating at post-tx.	CBT superior in early (by week 6) improvement (reduction in frequency of vomit episodes)
Garner et al., 1993[278] CBT vs. supportive-expressive therapy Outpatient Fair	Eating: • Binge episodes • EAT • EDE • EDI • Vomiting Biomarker: • Weight Psych: • BDI • Millon Inventory • RSE • SCL-90-R	No statistics reported.	No statistics reported.	Over 18 week tx period, CBT superior in reducing dieting, food preoccupation, eating concerns, restraint, attitudes toward shape, bulimia behaviors, depressed mood, global symptoms, and symptoms of borderline personality disorder and dysthymia; and in improving self-esteem.

Table 16. Results from behavioral intervention trials: bulimia nervosa (continued)

Source, Treatment, Setting, and Quality Score	Major Outcome Measures	Significant Change Over Time Within Groups	Significant Differences Between Groups at Endpoint	Significant Differences Between Groups in Change Over Time
Hsu et al., 2001[280] CT vs. NT vs. CT+NT (CNT) vs. group support (control) Outpatient Fair	Eating: • Bingeing • EDI • Meals/ week • Purging Psych: • HDRS	No statistics reported.	No statistics reported.	CNT superior to NT alone and to group support in binge/purge abstinence and in reducing drive for thinness and BN symptoms. CT superior to NT in reducing BN symptoms and CT superior to group support in reducing drive for thinness.
Sundgot-Borgen et al., 2002[283] Exercise vs. CBT vs. nutrition counseling vs. waiting-list vs. healthy controls Outpatient Fair	Eating: • Binge frequency • EDI • Vomit frequency • Laxative abuse Biomarker: • Percent body fat	Exercise group decreased percent body fat at post-tx and fat mass at 18-month FU.	Body dissatisfaction lower in CBT compared to nutritional counseling group at post tx. Laxative use lower in exercise than CBT group at post tx. Vomit frequency, bulimia symptoms, and body dissatisfaction lower in CBT than nutritional counseling group at 6 month FU. Drive for thinness and laxative abuse lower in exercise than CBT group, at 6 month FU. Binge episodes lower in exercise than in CBT at 18 month FU.	No statistics reported.
Chen et al., 2003[273] Individual CBT vs. group CBT Outpatient Fair	Eating: • Abstinence • Binge episodes • EDE-12 • Laxative use • Over-exercising • Purge episodes Biomarker: • BMI Psych: • BDI • SCL-90 • STAI	No statistics reported.	Higher rate of abstinence in individual CBT than group CBT at end of tx.	Group CBT superior to individual CBT in reducing state anxiety.

Table 16. Results from behavioral intervention trials: bulimia nervosa (continued)

Source, Treatment, Setting, and Quality Score	Major Outcome Measures	Significant Change Over Time Within Groups	Significant Differences Between Groups at Endpoint	Significant Differences Between Groups in Change Over Time
Agras et al., 1989[266] Waiting-list vs. Self-monitoring vs. CBT vs. CBT+ response prevention Outpatient Fair	Eating: • Abstinence • Dieting urge • Food preoccupation • Purge/week Biomarker: • Weight Psych: • BDI	Decreased purges/week in self-monitoring, CBT, and CBT+ response groups at end of 4-month tx.	CBT associated with higher abstinence rate compared to waiting-list at end of tx, and compared to self-monitoring and response prevention at 6 month FU.	CBT alone superior to waiting-list in reducing purging frequency, increasing purging abstinence and decreasing depressed mood, by end of treatment. CBT alone and CBT+ response prevention superior to waiting-list in reducing depressed mood by end of treatment.
Bulik et al., 1998;[270] Bulik et al., 1998;[271] Carter, McIntosh et al., 2003[272] 8 weeks CBT followed by B-ERP tx vs. P-ERP tx vs. relaxation training Outpatient Good	Eating: • Abstinence • Bingeing • Clinician ratings (food restriction, body dissatisfaction • EDI • Laxative use • Purging • Vomiting Psych: • HDRS • GAFS • SUDS	P-ERP and relaxation groups improved body dissatisfaction at 3 yr FU	B-ERP associated with less drive for thinness, lower clinician-rated food restriction, body dissatisfaction, and depressed mood, lower subjective distress than relaxation training at 3 year FU. P-ERP associated with fewer ED psychological and behavioral measures.than relaxation training at 3 year FU. B-ERP associated with less food restriction, higher GAFS score than relax training at 12 month FU.	Relaxation superior to B-ERP in reducing depressed mood and clinician-rated body dissatisfaction from post-tx to 2 year FU. Relaxation superior to P-ERP in reducing ED psych and behavioral traits and depressed mood from post-tx to 3 year FU.
Laessle et al., 1991[281] Nutritional management vs. stress management Outpatient Fair	Eating: • Binge frequency • Calories/day • EAT • EDI • Vomit frequency Psych: • BDI • STAI	No statistics reported.	No difference on any measures.	Nutritional management superior to stress management in increasing calorie consumption and decreasing binge frequency over first 3 weeks of tx, and in increasing binge abstinence rate through 6 and 12 months. Stress management superior to nutrition management in reducing trait anxiety over 3 months of tx.

Table 16. Results from behavioral intervention trials: bulimia nervosa (continued)

Source, Treatment, Setting, and Quality Score	Major Outcome Measures	Significant Change Over Time Within Groups	Significant Differences Between Groups at Endpoint	Significant Differences Between Groups in Change Over Time
Safer et al., 2001[282] DBT vs. waiting-list Outpatient Good	Eating: Binge episodes EDE Emotional eating scale Purge episodes Psych: BDI Positive and Negative Affect Schedule	No statistics reported.	DBT superior in post-tx abstinence rate	DBT superior in reducing the number of binge and purge episodes measured in last 4 of 20 weeks of tx.

only,[274] and by exploring the additive efficacy of exposure with response prevention grafted onto a basis of cognitive therapy.[271] Exposure with response prevention is defined as exposing individuals to their high-risk cues (e.g., prebinge cues or prepurge cues) and then preventing the response (e.g., binge eating or purging) until the urge to engage in the behavior subsides.

In comparisons of individually administered CBT and IPT tailored for BN, CBT was associated with a significantly greater probability of remission than IPT[269] and with greater decreases in vomiting and restraint[269,276] and binge eating[269] at the end of treatment. In one study at 1-year followup, these differences were no longer apparent.[276] Neither CBT nor IPT led to greater improvements in mood or changes in weight. Changes in dietary restraint and in eating self-efficacy mediated change in binge and purge frequency.[288] Being in the precontemplation stage of change was associated with failure to achieve remission at the end of treatment.[268]

When administered in group format, differences between CBT and IPT were less clear. Both group-administered treatments led to significantly greater decreases than waiting list on days binged, psychological features of the eating disorder, disinhibition, and restraint, with no differences observed between the active therapies.[287]

When compared directly, few differences emerged between group and individual administration of CBT. Both showed decreases in objective and subjective binge episodes, vomiting, laxative use, overexercise and EDI bulimia, drive for thinness, and body dissatisfaction subscale scores.[273] Group CBT was associated with greater decreases in anxiety; individual CBT was associated with significantly higher rates of abstinence. From a cost-effectiveness perspective, the study concluded that group CBT was more economical, given the similarity of outcomes.

In the dismantling studies, which attempted to parse out the effects of various components of CBT, the cognitive component emerged as critical to therapeutic outcome. Complete CBT led to better eating-related outcomes than BT,[276] to lower relapse than exposure with response prevention only,[274] and to greater abstinence than a self-monitoring only intervention.[266]

Two studies examined the additive efficacy of exposure with response prevention. Agras and colleagues found no additive benefit of exposure to CBT.[266] Bulik et al. first treated all patients with a core of cognitive therapy and then explored the added efficacy of three augmentation strategies: exposure with response prevention to prebinge cues, exposure with response prevention to prepurge cues, and a relaxation therapy control.[270] They found no evidence that either exposure treatment led to greater improvement in binge eating and vomiting than the relaxation control.

In other comparisons, cognitive therapy performed better than support only; adding a cognitive component to nutritional counseling led to a significantly greater decrease in drive for thinness than nutritional therapy alone.[280] CBT was superior to nutritional counseling alone in improving core binge eating, vomiting, laxative use, and body dissatisfaction. CBT also led to significantly greater decreases than supportive-expressive therapy (a nondirective psychodynamically oriented treatment) in EDI bulimia, EAT scores, food preoccupation, eating concerns, and depression.[278] Exercise therapy was superior to CBT at 18-month followup in improving drive for thinness, laxative abuse, and binge eating.[283]

Overall, dropout from CBT delivered individually or in group format ranged from 6 percent to 37 percent. Typical rates were about one-quarter of individuals randomized.

Other behavioral interventions. A single study compared nutritional management (focusing on decreasing restraint, detailed nutritional self-monitoring, and stimulus control) to stress management (focusing on decreasing stressors that may trigger binge eating). Both treatments led to significant decreases in binge eating and vomiting; abstinence from binge eating was greater in nutritional management than stress management, although abstinence from vomiting did not differ. Stress management was associated with greater reductions in trait anxiety.[281]

Dialectical behavioral therapy (DBT). DBT focuses on emotional dysregulation as the core problem in BN with symptoms viewed as attempts to manage unpleasant emotional states. A small study showed that patients receiving DBT had significantly greater decreases in binge eating and purging than did those on a waiting list and that abstinence was greater at the end of treatment in the DBT than in the waiting list group.[282]

Self-help trials. We present self-help trials for BN in Table 17. In a direct 18-week comparison of guided self-help (manual including visits with nonspecialists in eating disorders to check on progress) with group CBT, both treatments significantly decreased binge eating, vomiting, laxative use, EDI bulimia, drive for thinness and body dissatisfaction.[290] At 1-year followup, individuals in the self-help group showed greater reductions in vomiting and EDI bulimia. CBT was associated with greater reductions in drive for thinness over the treatment period and at followup. Both treatments significantly improved depression, with no differences between groups at the end of treatment; however, at followup, individuals in the self-help group had lower depression scores. Of those who completed treatment, a significantly greater number of individuals in the self-help group than in the CBT group were in remission for more than 2 weeks at the end of treatment (74 percent versus 44 percent). No significant change was seen in weight, although those in the self-help condition weighed significantly more at 1 year.

Carter et al. compared CBT-based self-help[302] with nonspecific self-help, focusing on self-assertion for women, with a waiting list control group in a 2-month trial.[291] Both self-help approaches led to significant decreases in objective binge episodes and purging; the waiting list did not. CBT-based self-help was associated with greater reductions in reducing intense exercise than nonspecific self-help or waiting list. No change in depression was observed. Abstinence and weight values were not reported.

To understand the feasibility and efficacy of self-help delivered in general practitioner (GP) offices, Durand and King compared GP-supported CBT-based self-help[303] with specialist outpatient treatment.[292] The duration of treatment was at the clinician's discretion. Patients in both groups reported significant decreases in scores on the Bulimic Investigation Test Edinburgh (BITE) and Eating Disorders Examination (EDE) total; however, binge eating and vomiting did

Table 17. Results from self-help trials, no medication: bulimia nervosa

Source, Treatment, Setting, and Quality Score	Major Outcome Measures	Significant Change Over Time Within Groups	Significant Differences Between Groups at Endpoint	Significant Differences Between Groups in Change Over Time
Bailer et al., 2004[290] Guided self-help vs. group CBT Outpatient Fair	Eating: • Binge frequency • EDI • Laxative use • Meal frequency • Recovery • Remittance • Vomit frequency Biomarker: • BMI Psych: • BDI	No statistics reported.	Higher meal frequency in self-help at post-tx. Lower vomit frequency, depressed mood, laxative use, and bulimia symptoms, and higher BMI in self-help, at 1-year FU.	Self-help superior to CBT in reducing bulimia symptoms over 18 weeks. CBT superior to self-help in reducing drive for thinness over tx and FU periods.
Carter et al., 2003[291] CBT-based self-help vs. non-specific self-help vs. waiting-list Outpatient Fair	Eating: • Binge frequency • EDE • Exercise frequency • Purge frequency Psych: • BAI • BDI • IIP	Both self-help groups decreased binge and purge frequencies. CBT-based self-help experienced a decrease in intense exercising.	No differences on any measures.	CBT-based self-help superior to non-specific self-help and to waiting-list in reducing intense exercising.
Durand and King, 2003[292] General practice physician- based self-help vs. specialist-based self-help Outpatient Fair	Eating: • BITE • Bulimic episodes • EDE • Vomit episodes Psych: • BDI • Patient-rated severity	No statistics reported.	No differences on any measures.	No differences on any measures.

BAI, Beck Anxiety Inventory; BDI, Beck Depression Inventory; BITE, Bulimic Investigation Text Edinborough; BMI, Body mass index; CBT, Cognitive Behavioral Therapy; EDE, Eating Disorder Examination; EDI, Eating Disorders Inventory; FU, followup; HDRS, Hamilton Depression Rating Scale [HDRS-17 items, HDRS-21 items]; IIP, Inventory of Interpersonal Problems; Psych, psychiatric and psychological; tx, treatment.

Table 17. Results from self-help trials, no medication: bulimia nervosa (continued)

Source, Treatment, Setting, and Quality Score	Major Outcome Measures	Significant Change Over Time Within Groups	Significant Differences Between Groups at Endpoint	Significant Differences Between Groups in Change Over Time
Thiels et al., 1998[293] CBT vs. guided self-change Outpatient Fair	Eating: • Binge abstinence • BITE • EDE • ED Awareness Test • Purge Abstinence Biomarker: • BMI Psych: • BDI • Self-esteem	No statistics reported.	Lower BITE scores in guided self-change group.	No differences on any measures.

not drop significantly. Both groups reported significant decreases in depression, but no treatment was superior. Weight change was not reported. Drop-out rates were similar across groups (24 percent in the GP group and 18 percent in specialist care).

A German study by Thiels et al. compared 16 weeks of CBT with guided self-change using a manual.[293] Guided self-change included 16 sessions with a therapist encouraging use of the manual and addressing motivation, obstacles, and emergent crises. Significant decreases occurred in overeating, vomiting, BITE scores, and EAT scores for both groups combined. Only on BITE scores did the CBT group perform significantly better than the guided self-change group. Depression dropped in both treatment groups with no significant differences between groups. Dropout was 13 percent in CBT and 29 percent in guided self-change.

Additional interventions for bulimia nervosa. We present other interventions for BN in Table 18. Three studies explored interventions that did not fit into our classification scheme: active light (such as that used to treat seasonal affective disorder), crisis prevention, and guided imagery.

Light therapy. In a small 8-week trial of 10,000 lux white light (active light) versus 50 lux red light (control), individuals in the active light group showed significantly greater decreases in binge eating than individuals in the control group.[295] Mood improved in both groups but no additional differences were observed for any other eating disorder, psychological, or biomarker outcome. The investigators did not provide long-term follow-up data. Given the size of this trial and the absence of followup, results should be viewed as preliminary.

Crisis prevention. Individuals who were abstinent after a trial of CBT were randomized to either a crisis prevention group in which they were able to contact their clinician to receive up to eight additional visits over 17 months if they felt their condition was deteriorating or a control follow-up-only group.[297] The percentage of individuals who resumed binge eating and purging did not differ over the 17-month interval; however, none of the individuals in the crisis prevention group used any of their available calls despite the reappearance of bulimic symptoms.

Table 18. Results from other trials: bulimia nervosa

Source, Treatment, Setting, and Quality Score	Major Outcome Measures	Significant Change Over Time Within Groups	Significant Differences Between Groups at Endpoint	Significant Differences Between Groups in Change Over Time
Braun et al., 1999[295] Bright light therapy vs. dim light/placebo Outpatient Fair	Eating: • Binge frequency • Meal frequency • Purge frequency • Seasonal patterns assessment questionnaire • YBC-EDS Psych: • BDI • HAM-D	No statistics reported.	No differences on any measures.	Bright light superior to dim light (placebo) in reducing binge frequency over 3 week tx.
Mitchell et al., 2004[297] Crisis prevention vs. usual follow-up Outpatient Fair	Eating: • Resumption of bingeing and/or purging after period of abstinence	No differences on any measures.	No differences on any measures.	No differences on any measures.
Esplen et al., 1998[296] Guided imagery vs. control (eating behavior journaling therapies) Outpatient Fair	Eating: • Abstinence • Binge frequency • EAT-26 • EDI • Purge frequency	No statistics reported.	Higher abstinence rate in guided imagery compared to control group.	Guided imagery superior to control in reducing binge and purge frequencies, drive for thinness, bulimia symptoms, and body dissatisfaction over 6 week tx period.

BDI, Beck Depression Inventory; EAT, Eating Attitudes Test (EAT-26 items); EDI, Eating Disorders Inventory; HAM-D, Hamilton Depression Rating Scale; Psych, psychiatric and psychological; tx, treatment; YBC-EDS, Yale-Brown-Cornell Eating Disorder Scale

Guided imagery. Esplen et al. conducted a 6-week trial of patients in a guided imagery group and a control journaling group.[296] Guided imagery was based on developing self-comforting in BN.[304] Guided imagery led to a significantly greater decrease in measures of binge eating, purging, EDI bulimia, drive for thinness, and body dissatisfaction. At the end of treatment, 21 percent of individuals in guided imagery and no individuals in the control condition were abstinent. Drop-out rates were comparable across groups.

Summary of behavioral interventions for bulimia nervosa. A large number of fair- to good-rated trials provide evidence that CBT administered individually or in group format is effective in reducing the core behavioral symptoms of binge eating and purging and psychological features of BN in both the short and the long term. One study suggests that CBT leads to more rapid reduction of symptoms than IPT.[276] Another suggests that individual CBT confers no advantage over the more economical group CBT approach;[273] although this finding is important for service delivery, it requires replication. The cognitive component of CBT appears to be the active ingredient for change, as behavioral interventions alone are not as effective.[274,276] Exposure with response prevention, either alone or as an added component to a core of cognitive therapy, offers no additional therapeutic advantage to basic CBT.[270,272,274]

Adding a cognitive component to nutritional intervention led to greater effectiveness in one study,[280] and CBT led to better outcomes than a psychodynamically oriented supportive-expressive therapy.[278] Preliminary evidence suggests that DBT is effective and worth additional study for the treatment of BN.[282]

Four studies provided mixed evidence regarding the efficacy of self-help methods for BN. One German and one Austrian study provide support for guided self-help in comparison to group CBT[290] and individually administered CBT.[293] The nature of the self-help approach (CBT oriented versus nonspecific) did not lead to different outcomes.[291] Preliminary evidence from the United Kingdom indicates that GPs can successfully deliver self-help.[292] No self-help trials conducted in the United States met our inclusion criteria. Overall, especially in the absence of control conditions, few conclusions can be drawn regarding the efficacy of self-help approaches for BN. Moreover, the term self-help must be considered carefully as many of the interventions labeled self-help included considerable contact with providers.

One report yielded preliminary evidence for treating BN with light leading to some short-term decreases in binge eating.[295] One study provided some support for guided imagery compared to journaling, although long-term maintenance of treatment effects is unknown.[296] Crisis prevention approaches do not appear to be effective in the treatment of BN, based on one study, as patients do not avail themselves of the opportunity to contact their therapists when symptoms reemerge.[297]

Key Question 2: Harms of Treatment for Bulimia Nervosa

Table 19 presents adverse events associated with treatments for BN. As reported in Chapter 3, harms from second-generation antidepressants include the following: for fluoxetine, insomnia, nausea, asthenia, tremor, dizziness, rhinitis, sweating, urinary frequency, and sexual dysfunction; for fluvoxamine, nausea, dizziness and drowsiness.[243] Adverse events associated with second-generation antidepressants in BN appear to be consistent with those observed in other disorders.[253]

Side effects of MAOI administration were nausea, sleep disturbance, and dizziness. No hypertensive crises were reported, although this danger should always be considered in patients who experience uncontrollable eating episodes.[121]

Key Question 3: Factors Associated With Treatment Efficacy

Medication Trials

A few medication trials for BN explored factors associated with outcome. Walsh et al. reported that patients with greater concern for body shape and weight and longer duration of illness had more favorable treatment responses.[257] The Fluoxetine BN Collaborative Study group found that heavier patients had higher response rates in each treatment group.[249]

Table 19. Adverse events reported: bulimia nervosa trials

Intervention	Adverse Event *†
Medication Trials	
Fluoxetine vs. placebo[244]	Fluoxetine group: Insomnia, nausea, and shakiness significantly more common Placebo group: depression more common
Fluoxetine vs. placebo[248]	Fluoxetine: significantly more trembling than placebo
Fluoxetine 60mg (F60) vs. fluoxetine 20mg (F20) vs. placebo (PL)[249]	Side effects by treatment group: Insomnia: F60 (30); F20 (23); PL (10); ($P < 0.001$) Nausea: F60 (28); F20 (20); PL (14); ($P = 0.021$) Asthenia: F60 (23); F20 (16); PL (11); ($P = 0.039$) Tremor: F60 (12); F20 (4); PL (0); ($P < 0.001$) Sweating: F60(7); F20 (4); PL (1); ($P = 0.036$) Urinary frequency: F60 (5); F20 (0); PL (2); ($P = 0.012$) Palpitation: F60(5); F20(1); PL(1); ($P = 0.017$) Yawn: F60 (5); F20(1); PL(1); ($P = 0.017$) Mydriasis: F60 (3); F20 (0); PL(0); ($P = 0.018$) Vasodilation: F60(1); F20 (4); PL (0); ($P = 0.029$)
Fluoxetine (F) vs. placebo (PL)[250]	Side effects by treatment group: Insomnia: F (102); PL (19); ($P < 0.05$) Nausea: F (90); PL(13); ($P < 0.001$) Asthenia, F (63); PL (7); ($P < 0.001$) Anxiety: F (52); PL (9); ($P < 0.05$) Tremor: F (42); PL (2); ($P < 0.001$) Dizziness: F (37); PL (4); ($P < 0.05$) Yawning, F (36); PL (0); ($P < 0.001$) Sweating: F (28); PL (2); ($P < 0.05$) Decreased libido: F (19); PL (1); ($P < 0.05$) Depression: F (30); PL (19); ($P < 0.05$) Myalgia: F (14); PL (12); ($P < 0.05$) Emotional lability: F (8); PL (8); ($P < 0.05$) Conjunctivitis: F (1); PL (3); ($P < 0.05$)
Fluoxetine vs. placebo[252]	Fluoxetine: hand tremor (5) Placebo: Palpitations (1)
Fluoxetine vs. placebo[254]	Fluoxetine: rhinitis (24) Placebo: rhinitis (12); ($P < 0.04$)
Fluvoxamine vs. placebo[247,299]	Fluvoxamine: nausea, dizziness and drowsiness significantly more common in patients receiving fluvoxamine Fluvoxamine: Drop outs due to general side effects (8)
Trazodone vs placebo[255]	Trazodone significantly more dizziness and drowsiness than placebo
Topiramate vs. placebo[251,259]	Topiramate: Dropouts (1) facial rash and irritability Placebo: Dropouts (2)
Brofaromine vs. placebo[253]	Brofaromine: nausea (2); sleep disturbance, nausea, dizziness Placebo: headache (1); dry mouth, nausea
Ondansetron vs. placebo[246]	No adverse events observed
Desipramine vs. placebo[257]	NR

CBT, cognitive behavioral therapy; DBT, dialectical behavioral therapy; NR: not reported
* If no numbers appear in parentheses, authors had only listed adverse events but not reported the number of cases.
† P values indicate differences between groups; they are reported with they are provided by the author.

Table 19. Adverse events reported: bulimia nervosa trials (continued)

Intervention	Adverse Event *†
Medication plus Behavioral Intervention Trials	
Fluoxetine vs. individual CBT vs. fluoxetine and individual CBT[261]	Fluoxetine: Dropouts due to side effects (4) Fluoxetine plus CBT: Dropouts due to side effects (2) Nature of side effects NR
Fluoxetine vs. manual based self-help[262]	NR
Fluoxetine plus guided self-help vs. placebo plus guided self help vs. fluoxetine vs. placebo[265]	NR
Desipramine 16 wks vs. despiramine 24 wks vs. desipramine 16 wks plus CBT vs. CBT only[260,300]	NR
Interpersonal psychotherapy vs. antidepressant (fluoxetine replaced by desipramine if no effect) in CBT nonresponders[263]	NR
CBT plus medication vs. CBT plus placebo vs. Supportive therapy plus med vs. supportive therapy plus placebo[264,301]	NR
Behavioral Intervention Trials	
CBT vs. Interpersonal psychotherapy[269]	9 withdrawn from treatment: 7 severe depression, 1 acute onset of panic disorder
CBT vs. exposure response prevention[274]	NR
CBT vs. Behavior therapy vs. interpersonal psychotherapy[267,276,277]	Behavior therapy: Drop out (1) severe weight loss
Group CBT vs. group Interpersonal psychotherapy vs. waiting list control[287]	NR
CBT vs. interpersonal psychotherapy[288]	NR
CBT vs. supportive-expressive therapy[278]	NR
Cognitive therapy vs. nutritional therapy[280]	NR
CBT vs. physical exercise vs. nutritional counseling[283]	Exercise: injury (1)
Individual CBT vs. Group CBT[273]	Alcohol abuse (2), AN (1), visual hallucinations (1). No indication of which group these participants were in.
CBT vs. CBT plus response prevention vs. self-monitoring vs. waiting-list[266]	NR
CBT plus exposure with response prevention to pre-binge cues vs. CBT plus exposure to response prevention with pre-purge cues vs. CBT plus relaxation training[270-272]	NR
Nutritional management vs. stress management[281]	NR
DBT vs. waiting list[282]	NR
Self-help Trials	
Guided self-help vs. group CBT[290]	NR
Self-help manual vs. waiting list control[291]	NR
Self-help intervention vs. clinic intervention[292]	NR
CBT vs. guided self-change sessions[293]	NR
Other Trials	
Active light vs. placebo dim light[295]	No adverse events observed
Crisis prevention vs. follow up[297]	NR
Guided imagery vs. control[296]	NR

Behavioral Intervention Trials

Behavioral interventions in BN provided better and reasonably consistent information about factors associated with treatment response. Several investigators reported two factors as associated with poor outcome: high frequency of binge eating[270,272,274,298,301] and longer duration of illness.[274,298]

Evidence was mixed or contradictory for other factors. Higher body dissatisfaction was associated with both poorer[270] and better outcome.[277] With respect to weight, a history of obesity was reported as a positive prognostic indicator[270] and as a predictor of dropout.[278] Better outcomes or more rapid response were associated with higher baseline depression, lower severity of binge eating,[287] and greater attitudinal disturbance at baseline.[277] Positive response was reported to be associated with a history of obesity, a history of alcoholism, and high scores for self-directedness[270] and self-control.[280] Poorer outcomes were associated with greater food restriction, higher depression, higher drive for thinness and bulimia scores on the EDI, and greater cue reactivity,[270] low self-esteem,[277] and precontemplation stage of change.[268]

Self-help Trials

Factors associated with positive response to self help included higher EDI perfectionism scores, higher Dimensional Assessment of Personality Pathology (DAPP) compulsivity scores, higher DAPP intimacy problem scores, and lower cognitive behavior knowledge scores.[291]

Other Interventions Trials

Higher soothing receptivity and ability to tolerate aloneness were associated with more positive outcomes in guided imagery therapy.[296]

Key Question 4: Treatment Efficacy by Subgroups

The total number of individuals enrolled in the 18 trials of drugs or drug plus behavioral interventions was 1,941. Of those 67 were men. No studies reported differential outcome by age. Thirteen studies failed to report the race or ethnicity of participants. Of those that did, 793 participants were identified as white, 57 as nonwhite, 33 as Asian, 12 as Hispanic American, and eight as African American. Of the 18 trials, 12 were conducted in the United States. No study analyzed results separately by sex or by race or ethnicity. Based on these results, we conclude that no information exists regarding differential efficacy of medication only or combined medication plus behavioral interventions for BN by sex, gender, age, race, ethnicity, or cultural group.

The total number of individuals enrolled in behavioral intervention or other intervention trials was 1,462. Of those, two were men. Of the 18 trials, 14 failed to reported race or ethnicity of participants. From the remaining four trials, 410 subjects were identified as white; 22 as nonwhite; 28 Hispanic-American; 26 as Asian; Maori or Pacific Islander; 19 as African-American or Afro-Caribbean; and one as Native American. In no instance did the investigators analyze results separately by race or ethnic group. No data exist regarding differential efficacy of behavioral interventions for BN by sex, gender, age, race, ethnicity, or cultural group.

Chapter 5. Results: Binge Eating Disorder

This chapter presents results of our literature search and our findings for the four key questions (KQs) pertaining to binge eating disorder (BED). KQ 1 sought evidence for the efficacy of various treatments or combinations of treatments for BED. KQ 2 sought evidence of harms associated with the treatment or combination of treatments for BED. KQ 3 addressed factors associated with the efficacy of treatment for BED. KQ 4 addressed whether the efficacy of treatment for BED differs by sex, gender, age, race, ethnicity, or cultural groups. We report first on specific details about the yields of the literature searches and characteristics of the studies, then on literature pertaining to treatment (KQ 1, KQ 2, and KQ 3). Summary tables presenting findings grouped by selected outcomes appear at the end of this chapter.

Overview of Included Studies

For each included BED study, detailed evidence tables appear in Appendix C.[††] We report first on medication trials (Evidence Table 10), then combined medication and behavioral interventions (Evidence Table 11), behavioral interventions only (Evidence Table 12), self-help interventions (Evidence Table 13), and other interventions (Evidence Table 14). Within each table, studies are listed alphabetically by author. For each study we report eating disorder-related outcomes, psychiatric and psychological outcomes (such as comorbid depression and anxiety), and biomarker outcomes including weight loss.

We identified 26 studies addressing treatment efficacy for BED. Nine were medication-only trials.[305-313] We rated four of these trials as good,[305,307,309,312] and five as fair.[306,308,310,311,313] One study of a medication no longer available in the United States (d-fenfluramine) is not discussed here.[313] The medications studied included second-generation antidepressants,[305-309] tricyclic antidepressants,[310] an anticonvulsant,[311] sibutramine,[312] and d-fenfluramine.[313]

Four trials combined medication with behavioral interventions using second-generation antidepressants,[314,315] a tricyclic antidepressant,[316] and orlistat.[317] Of these, we rated two as good,[315,317] one as fair,[316] and one as poor.[314]

We identified eight behavioral-intervention-only studies. Of these, we rated one trial as good,[318] three as fair,[319-321] and four as poor.[322-325] Of the four fair or good studies, three used some form of cognitive behavioral therapy (CBT) in comparison to other interventions[318-320] and one used dialectical behavior therapy (DBT).[321]

Three trials investigated various self-help methods.[326-328] We rated one as good[326] and two, which report on the same sample at two points in time, as fair.[327,328] Finally, one trial involved exercise, rated as poor,[329] and another examined virtual reality therapy, rated as fair.[330]

Studies with a quality rating of "poor" are not discussed below. Reasons that these studies received this rating are presented in Table 20. Although each study was not deficient in all areas, the following are the most common concerns contributing to the low rating of studies: randomization (no description of protections against researchers' influence, a fatal flaw in approach or the approach not described), assessors not being blinded or their blinding status not described, adverse events not described, the statistical analysis not including or not reporting whether a power analysis was conducted, a lack of necessary controls for confounding, and results not reported using an intention-to-treat approach.

[††] Appendixes cited in this report are provided electronically at
http://www.ahrq.gov/downloads/pub/evidence/pdf/eatingdisorders/eatdis.pdf.

Table 20. Reasons for poor quality ratings and number of trials with poor ratings: binge eating disorder

Reasons Contributing to Poor Ratings	Types of Intervention, Number of Times Flaw Was Detected, and Citations
Research Aim	
Hypothesis not clearly described	Medication-only trials: 0
	Psychotherapy trials: 0
Study Population	
Characteristics not clearly described	Medication-only trials: 0
	Psychotherapy trials: 0
No specific inclusion or exclusion criteria	Medication-only trials: 0
	Psychotherapy trials: 0
Randomization	
Protections against influence not in place	Medication-only trial: 1[314]
	Psychotherapy trials: 3[322-324]
Approach not described	Medication-only trials: 0
	Psychotherapy trials: 1[324]
Whether randomization had a fatal flaw not known	Medication-only trials: 0
	Psychotherapy trials: 4[322-325]
Comparison group(s) not similar at baseline	Medication-only trials: 0
	Psychotherapy trials: 0
Blinding	
Study subjects	Medication-only trials: 1[314]
	Psychotherapy trials: 0
Investigators	Medication-only trials: 1[314]
	Psychotherapy trials: 0
Outcomes assessors	Medication-only trial: 1[314]
	Psychotherapy trials: 4[322-325]
Interventions	
Interventions not clearly described	Medication-only trials: 0
	Psychotherapy trials: 0
No reliable measurement of patient compliance	Medication-only trials: 0
	Psychotherapy trials: 2[322,323]
Outcomes	
Results not clearly described	Medication-only trials: 0
	Psychotherapy trials: 0
Adverse events not reported	Medication-only trials: 0
	Psychotherapy trials: 3[322-324]

Table 20. Reasons for poor quality ratings and number of trials with poor ratings: binge eating disorder (continued)

Reasons Contributing to Poor Ratings	Types of Intervention, Number of Times Flaw Was Detected, and Citations
	Statistical Analysis
Statistics inappropriate	Medication-only trials: 0
	Psychotherapy trials: 1[325]
No controls for confounding (if needed)	Medication-only trials: 0
	Psychotherapy trials: 2[323,325]
Intention-to-treat analysis not used	Medication-only trials: 0
	Psychotherapy trials: 3[323-325]
Power analysis not done or not reported	Medication-only trial: 1[314]
	Psychotherapy trials: 3[322-324]
	Results
Loss to followup 26% or higher or not reported	Medication-only trials: 0
	Psychotherapy trials: 1[325]
Differential loss to followup 15% or higher or not reported	Medication-only trials: 0
	Psychotherapy trials: 2[324,325]
Outcome measures not standard, reliable, or valid in all groups	Medication-only trials: 0
	Psychotherapy trials: 0
	Discussion
Results do not support conclusions, taking possible biases and limitations into account	Medication-only trials: 0
	Psychotherapy trials: 0
Results not discussed within context of prior research	Medication-only trials: 0
	Psychotherapy trials: 0
External validity: population not representative of US population relevant to these treatments	Medication-only trials: 0
	Psychotherapy trials: 0
Funding/sponsorship not reported	Medication-only trial: 1[314]
	Psychotherapy trials: 0

Participants

Of the 19 studies rated fair or good, 14 were conducted in the United States,[305-309,311,315-318,320,321,327,328] and one each in Brazil,[312] Germany,[319] Italy,[330] Switzerland,[310] and the United Kingdom.[326] Five studies failed to report the age of participants; of the remainder, all focused on individuals 18 years of age or older (range, 18 to 65 years). With respect to sex, 1,132 individuals participated in fair or good clinical trials (984 women and 87 men; for 61 subjects, sex was not reported).

Six studies failed to report the race or ethnicity of participants. Of those that did, 775 participants were identified as white, 48 as nonwhite, 20 as African American, 12 as Hispanic American, and one as Native American. Drop-out rates from treatment trials appear in Table 21.

Key Question 1: Treatment Efficacy

Medication-only Trials

We report eight randomized controlled double-blind trials of medications (Table 22).[305-312] A total of 413 individuals enrolled in medication-only trials. Based on studies that reported sex (all except one study),[311] 322 women and 25 men participated in medication-only BED trials. The number of participants in the medication trials ranged from 20 to 85. The age of participants ranged from 18 to 60 years. Five trials reported the race of participants: 234 individuals were reported to be white and 29 nonwhite. Six trials were conducted in the United States,[305-309,311] one in Brazil,[312] and one in Switzerland.[310]

Second-generation antidepressants. *Fluoxetine.* One trial compared fluoxetine (average dose 71.3 mg/day) with placebo in 60 individuals meeting the Diagnostic and Statistical Manual for Psychiatric Disorders-Version IV (DSM IV) criteria for BED with three or more binges per week for 6 months and higher than 85 percent ideal body weight (IBW) in a 6-week flexible dose trial.[305] Fluoxetine significantly decreased binges per week, severity of illness, and clinician-rated depression scores. It was associated with less weight gain than the placebo, although both groups gained weight during treatment. The investigators failed to report abstinence rates and long-term followup. Dropout was 57 percent in the fluoxetine group and 23 percent in the placebo group. Any inferences made from this study must be made with extreme caution because of the very high and differential attrition rate.

Other second-generation antidepressants. A 9-week trial compared fluvoxamine (50-300 mg/day) with placebo in 85 patients with BED, at least three binge eating episodes per week for 6 months, and higher than 85 percent of the midpoint of their ideal weight for height. Using intention-to-treat analyses, the investigators showed that patients on fluvoxamine had a significantly greater rate of reduction in binge frequency than those on placebo; however, the remission rate did not differ between groups.[306] The rate of improvement in severity of illness but not in depression was greater in the fluvoxamine group than in the placebo group. Fluvoxamine led to a greater rate of reduction of body mass index (BMI); however, BMI at endpoint was not reported so the clinical significance of the weight change could not be evaluated. The investigators failed to report long-term followup. Overall dropout was 21 percent.

In a 12-week trial of fluvoxamine (average dose 239 mg/day) versus placebo in 20 patients with DSM-IV BED, investigators observed no differences between fluvoxamine and placebo on binge eating frequency, although both groups combined showed decreases in binge frequency at the end of treatment.[307] Both groups combined had significant decreases in shape and weight concerns with no differences between them. Self-reported depression decreased similarly for both. Neither group showed significant weight change with treatment. The investigators failed to report long-term followup. Overall dropout was 20 percent.

McElroy et al. compared 6 weeks of sertraline (mean dose 187 mg/day) with placebo in 34 individuals with DSM-IV BED, at least three binge episodes per week for 6 months, and greater than 85 percent of IBW.[309] Sertraline led to greater reduction in binges per week but not with complete remission when rated categorically. It was also associated with increased reduction in

Table 21. Dropout rates for randomized controlled trials: binge eating disorder

Author	Total Enrollment, N	Total Dropouts, N (%)	G1 Treatment (% Dropout)	G2 Treatment (% Dropout)	G3 Treatment (% Dropout)	G4 Treatment (% Dropout)
Medication Trials						
Arnold et al., 2002[305]	60	24 (40%)	Fluoxetine (57%)	Placebo (23%)		
Hudson et al., 1998[306]	85	18 (21%)	Fluoxetine (NR)	Placebo (NR)		
Pearlstein et al., 2003[307]	25	5 (20%)	Fluvoxamine (NR)	Placebo (NR)		
McElroy et al., 2000[309]	34	8 (24%)	Sertaline (28%)	Placebo (19%)		
McElroy et al., 2003[308]	38	7 (18%)	Citalopram (16%)	Placebo (21%)		
Laederach-Hoffman et al., 1999[310]	31	2 (7%)	Imipramine (7%)	Placebo (6%)		
McElroy et al., 2003[311]	61	26 (43%)	Topiramate (47%)	Placebo (39%)		
Appolinario et al., 2003[312]	60	12 (20%)	Sibutramine (23%)	Placebo (17%)		
Medication plus Behavioral Intervention Trials						
Grilo, Masheb, and Wilson, 2005[315]	108	22 (20%)	Placebo (15%)	Fluoxetine (22%)	CBT + placebo (21%)	CBT + fluoxetine (23%)
Agras et al., 1994[316]	109	24 (22%)	Weight loss therapy (27%)	CBT + Weight loss (17%)	CBT + Weight loss + desipramine (23%)	
Grilo, Masheb, and Salant, 2005[317]	50	11 (22%)	Orlistat + CBT (24%)	Placebo + CBT (20%)		
Behavioral Interventions						
Gorin, Le Grange, and Stone, 2003[320]	94	32(34%)	Standard CBT (NR)	Standard CBT with spouse involvement (NR)	Waiting list control (NR)	
Hilbert and Tuschen-Caffier, 2004[319]	28	4 (14%)	CBT with a body exposure component (14%)	CBT with a cognitive restructuring component focused on body image (14%)		
Wilfley et al., 2002[318]	162	29 (18%)	CBT (20%)	Interpersonal psychotherapy (16%)		
Telch, Agras, and Linehan, 2001[321]	44	10 (23%)	Dialectical behavior therapy (18%)	Waiting list control (27%)		

CBT, cognitive behavioral therapy; G, group; N, number; NR, not reported.

Table 21. Dropout rates for randomized controlled trials: binge eating disorder (continued)

Author	Total Enrollment, N	Total Dropouts, N (%)	G1 Treatment (% Dropout)	G2 Treatment (% Dropout)	G3 Treatment (% Dropout)	G4 Treatment (% Dropout)
			Self-help			
Carter and Fairburn, 1998[326]	72	9 (12%)	Guided self-help (24%)	Pure self-help (0%)	Waiting list control (4%)	
Peterson et al., 1998[328]	50 (to active treatment)	8 (16%)	Therapist-led (13%)	Partial self-help (11%)	Structured self-help (27%)	Waiting list control (0%)
Peterson et al., 2001[327]	51	7 (14%)	Therapist-led (NR)	Partial self-help (NR)	Structured self-help (NR)	
Riva et al., 2002[330]	20	0 (0%)	Virtual Reality (0%)	Psych-nutritional group (0%)		

94

Table 22. Results from medication trials: binge eating disorder

Source, Treatment, Setting, and Quality Score	Major Outcome Measures	Significant Change Over Time Within Groups	Significant Differences Between Groups at Endpoint	Significant Differences Between Groups in Change Over Time
Arnold et al., 2002[305] Fluoxetine vs. placebo Outpatient Good	Eating: • Abstinence • Binge eating Biomarker: • BMI • Weight Psych: • CGI • HAM-D	No statistics reported	Fluoxetine associated with lower illness severity and depressed mood, and less weight gain.	Fluoxetine superior in reducing binge frequency, illness severity, and depressed mood, and in controlling weight and BMI gain over 6 weeks.
Hudson et al., 1998[306] Fluvoxamine vs. placebo Outpatient Fair	Eating: • Binge eating • Remission Biomarker: • BMI Psych: • CGI • HDRS	No statistics reported	No statistics reported	Fluvoxamine superior in reducing binge frequency, clinical severity, and BMI over 9 weeks.
Pearlstein et al., 2003[307] Fluvoxamine vs. placebo Outpatient Good	Eating: • Binge eating • EDE Biomarker: • Weight Psych: • BDI • HAM-D • SCL-90	No statistics reported	No statistics reported	No differences on any measures
McElroy et al., 2003[311] Topiramate vs. placebo Outpatient Fair	Eating: • Binge eating • YBOCS-BE Biomarker: • BMI • Weight Psych: • CGI • HDRS	No statistics reported	No statistics reported.	Topiramate superior in reducing binge frequency, illness severity, eating-related obsessions, compulsions, BMI, and weight over 14 weeks.

BDI, Beck Depression Inventory; BES, Binge Eating Scale; BMI, body mass index; CGI, Clinical Global Impressions; EDE, Eating Disorders Examination; FU, followup; HAM-D, Hamilton Depression Inventory; HDRS, Hamilton Depression Rating Scale; Psych, psychiatric and psychological; SCL-90, (Hopkins) Symptom Check List; SDS, Self-rating Depression Scale; vs., versus; YBOCS-BE, Yale-Brown Obsessive Compulsive Scale (modified for binge eating).

Table 22. Results from medication trials: binge eating disorder (continued)

Source, Treatment, Setting, and Quality Score	Major Outcome Measures	Significant Change Over Time Within Groups	Significant Differences Between Groups at Endpoint	Significant Differences Between Groups in Change Over Time
McElroy et al., 2003[308] Citalopram vs. placebo Outpatient Fair	Eating: • Binge eating • YBOCS-BE Biomarker: • BMI • Weight Psych: • CGI • HAM-D	No statistics reported	Citalopram asscociated with greater reduction in frequency of binge days, BMI, and weight.	Citalopram superior to placebo in the rate of reduction in frequency of binges, illness severity, binge eating related obsessions and compulsions, and weight over 6 weeks.
Laederach-Hoffman et al., 1999[310] Imipramine vs. placebo (with dietary and psychological counseling Outpatient Fair	Eating: • Binge eating Biomarker: • BMI • Waist-hip ratio weight Psych: • HAM-D • SDS	Imipramine decreased binge frequency and depressed mood over 8 weeks, and decreased depressed mood and weight at 32 week FU.	No statistics reported	Imipramine superior to placebo in decreasing binge frequency, depressed mood, and body weight over 8 weeks of active tx, and 32-week FU.
McElroy, Casuto et al., 2000[309] Sertraline vs. placebo Outpatient Good	Eating: • Binge eating Biomarker: • BMI Psych: • CGI • HDRS	No statistics reported	No statistics reported	Sertraline superior to placebo in reducing binge frequency, illness severity, and BMI, and in increasing global improvement over 6 weeks.
Appolinario et al., 2003[312] Sibutramine hydrochloride vs. placebo Outpatient Good	Eating: • BES • Binge eating • Remission Biomarker: • Weight Psych: • BDI	No statistics reported	Sibutramine associated with less depressed mood.	Sibutramine superior to placebo in reducing binge frequency and severity. Difference in weight at end of treatment with weight decreasing over treatment period in the sibutramine group but increasing in the placebo group.

severity of illness but not with depression scores. The drug also led to greater reductions in weight; however, the investigators failed to report BMI at endpoint so the clinical significance of the weight change is unclear. The investigators failed to present long-term follow-up data. Dropout was 28 percent in the sertraline group and 19 percent in the placebo group.

In a 6-week trial of citalopram (40-60 mg/day) versus placebo in 38 individuals with BED, with three or more binge episodes per week for 6 months and more than 85 percent of IBW, the active drug led to a significantly greater rate of decrease of binge eating and binge eating days; however, the percentage of individuals remitted when measured categorically did not differ significantly.[308] The citalopram group showed greater reductions in clinician-rated obsession and compulsion scores and in severity of illness and depression scores. The BMI rate of change was significantly greater in the citalopram group; patients lost on average 2.7 kg and those on placebo gained 5.2 kg during treatment. Although the rate of change data suggested more rapid response in the citalopram group, differences between the groups over time were not significant for the core outcome variables of binges per week or severity of illness. Dropout was 16 percent in the citalopram group and 21 percent in the placebo group.

Tricyclic antidepressants. Laederach-Hoffman et al. augmented standard bi-weekly diet counseling and psychological support with either impiramine (25 mg three times a day) or placebo in 31 individuals with DSM-IV BED and BMI greater than 27.5.[310] Significantly greater reductions in binge eating episodes and Hamilton Depression Rating Scale (HAM-D) scores occurred in the impiramine group at 8 and 32 weeks. Body weight was significantly reduced in the imipramine group at 8 and 32 weeks (mean reduction of 2.1 kg at 8 weeks and 5.0 kg at 32 weeks); the placebo group gained weight. Abstinence rates were not reported. Low doses of imipramine when delivered in the context of psychological support and diet counseling led to maintenance of decreased binge eating, depression, and weight. Dropout was between 6 percent and 7 percent in both groups.

Anticonvulsants. One 14-week trial compared topiramate (average dose 212 mg/day) with placebo in 61 individuals with BED, BMI greater than 30, and a score greater than 15 on the Yale-Brown Obsessive Compulsive Scale for Binge Eating (YBOCS-BE).[311] Patients receiving topiramate experienced a significantly greater rate of change and a significantly greater percentage reduction in binge episodes, binge days per week, and YBOC-BE. Severity of illness, but not depression scores, showed greater improvement in the topiramate group. Topiramate led to significantly greater and clinically meaningful weight loss (5.9 kg) than placebo (1.2 kg). No follow-up data were provided. The investigators failed to report abstinence rates or endpoint values, so estimating the magnitude of clinical significance of differences is difficult. Dropout was 47 percent in the topiramate group and 39 percent in the placebo group.

Sibutramine. A 12-week comparison of sibutramine (15 mg/day) with placebo in 60 individuals with DSM-IV BED and a Binge Eating Scale (BES) score of greater than or equal to 17 indicated that sibutramine produced significant decreases in binge days per week and BES scores than placebo.[312] Sibitramine was also associated with a significant decrease in self-reported depression scores over the course of treatment. At week 12, the sibutramine group had lost on average 7.4 kg whereas the placebo group gained weight (a significant difference). The authors did not report abstinence rates or provide long-term follow-up data. Dropout was 23 percent in the sibutramine group and 17 percent in the placebo group.

Summary of medication-only trials. Treating BED in overweight individuals has two critical outcomes—decrease in binge eating and decrease in weight. Although not all BED studies explicitly sampled on the basis of weight, all focused on overweight individuals. Four selective serotonin reuptake inhibitors (SSRIs)—one serotonin, dopamine, and norepinephrine uptake inhibitor; one tricyclic antidepressant; one anticonvulsant; and one appetite suppressant—have been studied in BED. In short-term trials, SSRIs appear to lead to greater rates of reduction in target eating, psychiatric and weight symptoms, and severity of illness. However, in the absence of clear endpoint data, and in the absence of data regarding abstinence from binge eating, we cannot judge the magnitude of the clinical impact of these interventions. Moreover, lacking follow-up data after drug discontinuation, we do not know whether observed changes in binge eating, depression, and weight persist.

Low-dose imipramine as an augmentation strategy to standard dietary counseling and psychological support is associated with decreases in binge eating and weight that persist after discontinuation of the medication. This finding suggests a potentially promising pairing worth further investigation.

Both sibutramine and topiramate yielded promising results in terms of weight reduction for patients with BED: clinically significant reductions in BMI over the short term. The authors of these reports did not supply remission rates. Additional research is required to track patients after drug discontinuation to determine whether observed changes in eating behavior and weight persist.

Several studies reported rate of change of symptoms rather than actual differences in groups in change over time including endpoint values. Although rate of change is of interest, endpoint measures, including consistently defined abstinence rates, are critical to evaluate the clinical status of participants at the end of treatment.

Overall, drop-out rates were between 16 percent and 57 percent in the medication trials for BED. The high placebo response in BED is noteworthy.

Medication Plus Behavioral Intervention Trials

We present three trials of medications plus psychotherapy in Table 23.[315-317] The total number of individuals enrolled in these combination trials was 267 (237 women and 30 men).

The number of participants in these combination trials ranged from 50 to 109. Age ranged from 21 to 65 years. Of these three trials, two reported the race or ethnicity of participants: 140 individuals were reported as white, 12 as African American, and six as Hispanic American.[315,317] The United States was the site of all three trials.

Second-generation antidepressants and CBT. Grilo et al. compared fluoxetine (60 mg/day) with placebo, both with and without CBT, in a 16-week trial.[315] Treatment groups receiving CBT reported greater reductions in binge episodes, eating and shape concerns, disinhibition, and depression and greater remission rates than did the medication-only or placebo groups. Weight loss did not differ across groups; the authors did not report within-group weight loss over time. Dropout between groups was comparable (between 15 percent and 23 percent).

Tricyclic antidepressants and CBT. Agras et al. compared the effects of weight-loss treatment, CBT, and desipramine in 109 individuals with DSM IV BED. They randomly allocated participants to 9 months of weight-loss-only therapy, 3 months of CBT followed by 6 months of weight-loss therapy, or 3 months of CBT followed by 6 months of weight-loss therapy and desipramine (300 mg/day).[316] Groups receiving CBT showed significant reduction in binge eating at 12 weeks but not at any later follow-up point. Likewise, any observed differences on self-report measures of eating pathology were no longer significantly different at 36 weeks. Changes in depression scores did not differ across groups. Initial weight loss was greater in the weight-loss therapy group. At 3-month followup, the greatest weight loss was seen in the group including CBT and desipramine (average reduction of 4.8 kg from baseline). Dropout from acute treatment was comparable across groups: from 27 percent in the weight-loss therapy group to 17 percent in the CBT plus weight-loss therapy group.

Orlistat and CBT. In a 12-week trial of orlistat (120 mg three times/day) with CBT and placebo with CBT in 50 individuals with DSM-IV BED and BMI > 30, the orlistat group had greater remission rates at the end of treatment but not at 2-month followup.[317] The authors reported no differences in any other eating-related or depression measures. Individuals in the orlistat group experienced greater initial weight loss (-3.5 kg) than those in the placebo group

Table 23. Results from medication plus behavioral intervention trials: binge eating disorder

Source, Treatment, Setting, and Quality Score	Major Outcome Measures	Significant Change Over Time Within Groups	Significant Differences Between Groups at Endpoint	Significant Differences Between Groups in Change Over Time
Grilo, Masheb, Salant, 2005[317] CBT + orlistat vs. CBT + placebo Outpatient Good	Eating: • EDE • Remission Biomarker: • Weight loss Psych: • BDI	No statistics reported	Greater percentage of CBT + orlistat group remitted and achieved at least 5 percent weight loss over 12 weeks. Group difference in weight loss maintained at 2-month FU	CBT + orlistat superior in total weight loss and in percent weight loss to post-tx over 12 weeks.
Agras et al., 1994[316] Weight loss therapy vs. CBT+weight loss therapy vs. CBT+weight loss therapy + desipramine Outpatient Fair	Eating: • Binge eating • TFEQ Biomarker: • Weight Psych: • BDI	No statistics reported	No statistics reported	CBT plus weight loss (with or without desipramine) superior to weight loss alone in reducing binge frequency over 12 weeks. Significant difference between groups at 12 wks in change in weight over time with weight decreasing in weight loss group and increasing in CBT groups. By 3 month FU, CBT plus desipramine superior to CBT without desipramine in reducing weight.
Grilo, Masheb, Wilson, 2005[315] Fluoxetine vs. placebo vs. CBT + placebo vs. CBT + fluoxetine Outpatient Good	Eating: • Binge eating • BSQ • EDE • Remission • TFEQ Biomarker: • BMI Psych: • BDI	No statistics reported	No statistics reported	CBT groups superior to placebo and fluoxetine alone in decreasing binge frequency, eating and shape concerns, global eating score, disinhibition, and rate of remission. CBT + fluoxetine superior to placebo alone and fluoxetine alone in decreasing weight concerns and hunger; superior to fluoxetine alone in reducing depressed mood and dietary restraint; superior to placebo in decreasing body dissatisfaction. CBT + placebo superior to placebo alone and fluoxetine alone in decreasing depressed mood; superior to fluoxetine alone in decreasing dietary restraint, weight concerns, and body dissatisfaction.

BDI, Beck Depression Inventory; BMI, Body mass index; BSQ, Body Shape Questionnaire; CBT, Cognitive Behavioral Therapy; EDE, Eating Disorders Examination; FU, followup; Psych, psychiatric and psychological; TFEQ, Three Factor Eating Questionnaire; Tx, treatment, vs., versus.

(-1.6 kg), but that loss was not maintained at followup; at followup, however, the orlistat group was more likely to have achieved a weight loss of 5 percent or more. Dropout (about 20 percent) was comparable between groups.

Summary of medication plus psychotherapy trials. Adding CBT conferred benefit on remission rate, but not weight loss, over fluoxetine alone or placebo alone in one trial.[315] Adding CBT to orlistat was associated with a greater decrease in weight during treatment, although this does not appear to be maintained at followup.[317] In one trial, adding desipramine to CBT and weight loss therapy led to greater maintenance of weight loss over time.[316] Combining medication and CBT may improve both binge eating and weight loss, although sufficient trialshave not been done to determine definitively which medications are best at producing and maintaining weight loss. Moreover, the optimal duration of medication treatment for sustained reductions in binge eating and maintenance of weight loss has not yet been addressed empirically.

Behavioral Intervention Trials

We identified eight behavioral intervention-only trials (Table 24),[318-325] three trials of self-help (Table 25),[326-328] and one trial each of exercise and virtual reality (Table 26).[329,330]

In behavioral intervention trials, CBT tailored for BED was the most commonly tested therapeutic approach; one study used DBT. The total number of individuals enrolled in psychotherapy, self-help, exercise, and virtual reality trials was 481 (449 women and 32 men). Of the eight trials identified, participants ranged in age from 18 to 65 years. Six trials reported the race and ethnicity of participants: in all, they involved 401 persons identified as white, 19 individuals as nonwhite, eight as African American or Afro-Caribbean, six as Hispanic American, one as Native American, and one as Asian. In no instance were results analyzed specifically by race or ethnic group. Of the eight trials, five were conducted in the United States and one each in Germany, the United Kingdom, and Italy.

Behavioral intervention trials for binge eating disorder. *CBT.* A 12-week trial of standard CBT tailored for BED compared with CBT and spousal involvement and with a waiting list control group in 94 individuals with a BMI of 25 or more showed that both active CBT groups had significant reductions in days binged, BMI, disinhibition, hunger, depression, and self-esteem than the controls and were more likely to be abstinent from binge eating at the end of treatment. Adding spousal involvement did not produce significantly greater improvements than standard CBT.[320] Both CBT groups had significantly lower depression scores and BMI, but they did not differ from each other. The average BMI decrease from baseline to followup was 0.11 for CBT and 0.77 for CBT with spousal involvement, suggesting that CBT alone, with or without a spouse participating, did not yield substantial weight change. Overall, dropout was 34 percent.

Hilbert et al. studied 5 months of group CBT with body exposure treatment and group CBT with cognitive restructuring of negative body cognitions in 28 women with BED, using a broad inclusion criterion of at least one binge per week.[319] Both groups showed decreases in binge eating, psychological aspects of binge eating, self-report binge eating scores, and decreases in self-report depression, but differences between groups were not statistically significant. Neither group experienced significant weight loss. Dropout was 14 percent in each group.

Looking at the efficacy of group psychotherapy, Wilfley et al. compared group CBT with group IPT in 20 sessions with 3 additional individual sessions in 162 individuals with BED and BMI levels between 27 and 48.[318] Both therapies led to significant decreases in the number of days binged at the end of treatment and at 4-month followup. CBT led to greater improvements in Eating Disorders Examination Restraint scores at all time points. At 12 months, the groups did not differ in abstinence (CBT, 72 percent; IPT, 70 percent), severity of illness, or depression; both treatments led to significant reductions in these parameters. No participants in either group

Table 24. Results from behavioral intervention trials, no medication: binge eating disorder

Source, Treatment, Setting, and Quality Score	Major Outcome Measures	Significant Change Over Time Within Groups	Significant Differences Between Groups at Endpoint	Significant Differences Between Groups in Change Over Time
Gorin et al., 2003[320] Group-based CBT vs. CBT with spouse involvement vs. waiting list Outpatient Fair	Eating: • Abstinence • Binge eating • TFEQ Biomarker: • BDI Psych: • BMI	No statistics reported	Higher percent abstinent in CBT groups compared to waiting list.	CBT (with and without spouse involvement) superior to waiting list in decreasing number of binge days, disinhibition, hunger, depressed mood, and BMI over 12 weeks.
Hilbert and Tuschen-Caffier, 2004[319] CBT+exposure vs. CBT+cognitive interventions for image disturbance Outpatient Fair	Eating: • Binge eating • Body Satisfaction • EDE • Negative automatic thoughts • Recovery Biomarker: • BMI Psych: • BDI	Binge frequency, depressed mood, shape and weight concerns, body dissatisfaction, and restraint decreased in both groups over time.	No differences in percent recovered.	No differences on any measures.
Wilfley et al., 2002[318] CBT vs. IPT Outpatient Good	Eating: • Abstinence • Binge eating • EDE Biomarker: • BMI Psych: • GSI • SCL-90	Both interventions associated with decreased number of binge days and eating restraint at post-tx, 4- and 8-month FU. Both tx associated with decreased GSI total scores; shape, weight, and eating concerns, restraint, and depressed mood at post-tx.	Less restraint in CBT at post-tx and 4-month FU.	CBT superior in decreasing eating restraint at post-tx and 4, 8, and 12 month FU.

BDI, Beck Depression Inventory; BES, Binge Eating Scale; BMI, body mass index; CBT, Cognitive Behavioral Therapy; DBT, Dialectical Behavior Therapy; EDE, Eating Disorders Examination; EES, Emotional Eating Scale; FU, followup; GSI, General Severity Index (derived from BSI); PANAS, Positive and Negative Affect Schedule; Psych, psychiatric and psychological; RSE, Rosenberg Self-Esteem Scale; SCL-90, (Hopkins) Symptom Check ListTFEQ, Three Factor Eating Questionnaire; Tx, treatment, vs. versus.

Table 24. Results from behavioral intervention trials, no medication: binge eating disorder

Source, Treatment, Setting, and Quality Score	Major Outcome Measures	Significant Change Over Time Within Groups	Significant Differences Between Groups at Endpoint	Significant Differences Between Groups in Change Over Time
Telch et al., 2001[321] DBT vs. waiting list Outpatient Fair	Eating: • BES • Binge eating • EDE • EES Biomarker: • Weight Psych: • BDI • PANAS • RSE	No statistics reported	No statistics reported	DBT superior to waiting list control in decreasing number of binge episodes and binge days, binge severity, and weight, shape, and eating concerns.

Table 25. Results from self-help trials, no medication: binge eating disorder

Source, Treatment, Setting, and Quality Score	Major Outcome Measures	Significant Change Over Time Within Groups	Significant Differences Between Groups at Endpoint	Significant Differences Between Groups in Change Over Time
Carter and Fairburn, 1998[326] Guided self-help vs. non-guided self-help vs. waiting list Outpatient Good	Eating: • Abstinence • Binge eating • EDE Biomarker: • BMI • Weight Psych: • BSI • GSI	Both self-help groups decreased binge eating, GSI, and EDE global at 12-week post-tx. Guided self-help only decreased eating restraint at post-tx.	Both self-help groups associated with higher abstinence rates, less binge eating, and lower GSI, EDE global and restraint scores, compared to waiting list at post-tx. Guided self-help associated with less restraint and binge eating at 3 month FU and with less binge eating at 6 month FU compared to non-guided self-help.	Guided self-help superior to non-guided self-help and waiting list in reducing eating restraint over 12 weeks.
Peterson et al., 1998[328] Therapist-led group CBT vs. partial self-help group CBT vs. structured self-help group CBT vs. waiting list Outpatient Fair	Eating: • Abstinence • BES • Binge eating • BSQ • Eating Behavior-IV • TFEQ Biomarker: • BMI Psych: • HDRS • RSE	No statistics reported	Abstinence rates for binge eating higher in each of the CBT groups compared to waiting list	CBT groups superior to waiting list in decreasing objective and total binge episodes/week, hours spent binge eating/week, binge severity, disinhibition, and hunger over 8 weeks.
Peterson et al., 2001[327] Therapist-led group CBT vs. partial self-help group CBT vs. structured self-help group CBT Outpatient Fair	Eating: • Abstinence • Binge eating • BSQ • TFEQ Biomarker: • BMI Psych: • BDI • HDRS	No statistics reported	Abstinence from total binge episodes higher in structured self-help group versus therapist-led self-help and partial self-help groups.	No differences on any measures

BDI, Beck Depression Inventory; BES, Binge Eating Scale; BMI, Body mass index; BSI, Brief Symptom Inventory; BSQ, Body Shape Questionnaire; CBT, Cognitive Behavioral Therapy; EDE, Eating Disorders Examination; FU, followup; GSI, General Severity Index (derived from BSI); HDRS, Hamilton Depression Rating Scale; Psych, psychiatric and psychological; RSE, Rosenberg Self-Esteem Scale; TFEQ, Three Factor Eating Questionnaire; Tx, treatment, vs., versus.

Table 26. Results from other trials: binge eating disorder

Source, Treatment, Setting, and Quality Score	Major Outcome Measures	Significant Change Over Time Within Groups	Significant Differences Between Groups at Endpoint	Significant Differences Between Groups in Change Over Time
Riva et al., 2002 Virtual reality-based tx for body image vs. CBT-based psycho-nutritional group therapy Inpatient Fair	Eating: • Abstinence • BIAQ • BSS • CDRS • DIET • FRS • WELSQ Psych: • STAI	Virtual reality tx associated with increased ideal body score and WELSQ total score, and decreased state anxiety.	No statistics reported	Virtual reality tx superior to psycho-nutritional tx in increasing WELSQ total score and in decreasing state anxiety and overeating.

BMI, Body mass index; BIAQ, Body Image Avoidance Questionnaire; BSS, Body Satisfaction Scale; CBT, cognitive behavioral therapy; CDRS, Contour Drawing Rating Scale; DIET, Dieter's Inventory of Eating Temptations; FRS, Figure Rating Scale; Psych, psychiatric and psychological; STAI, Spielberger State-Trait Anxiety Inventory; Tx, treatment; WELSQ, Weight Efficacy Life-style Questionnaire.

experienced reductions in BMI across treatment or follow-up periods. Dropout was 20 percent in CBT and 16 percent in IPT.

Dialectical behavioral therapy. Twenty weeks of DBT led to greater reduction in binge days, binge episodes, weight concern, shape concern, and eating concern than did being in a waiting list control group in 44 women with DSM-IV BED.[321] Depression and anxiety scores did not differ. The authors did not report whether DBT was associated with significant change in weight, although no differences in weight loss emerged between groups during treatment. Dropout was 18 percent in the DBT group and 55 percent in the waiting list group.

Self-help trials. Carter and Fairburn compared guided self-help using a book[302] combined with six to eight sessions with a facilitator with self-help-only using the same book in the absence of a facilitator and with waiting list controls in 72 women with BED with weekly binges.[326] Both self-help approaches were more efficacious than the control arm in reducing the mean number of binge days and improving abstinence and cessation rates and EDE scores. At the end of treatment, both self-help groups showed significantly greater reductions in clinical severity than the control group. No group reported significant weight loss at any point. Comparisons of the two self-help groups yielded no differences in eating, depression, or BMI measures at any follow-up point. Dropout was 24 percent from guided self-help and 4 percent from the control group; self-help-only had no dropouts.

In a four-group comparison, Peterson et al. compared therapist-led self-help, partial self-help, structured self-help, and waiting list controls in 61 individuals with DSM IV BED.[328] In therapist-led self-help, a doctoral-level therapist led both the psychoeducational component and group discussion; in the partial self-help group, participants viewed a 30-minute psychoeducational videotape and then participated in a therapist-led discussion; and in the structured self-help group, subjects viewed the 30-minute psychoeducational videotape and then led their own 30-minute discussion. All self-help groups performed better than controls on objective binges, total binges, hours spent bingeing, and self-reported eating attitudes. For abstinence rates, all self-help groups (68 percent to 87 percent) were better than controls (12.5 percent). The groups did not differ in depression scores or BMI changes. Dropout was higher in the structured self-help group (27 percent) than in the therapist-led (13 percent) and partial (11 percent) self-help groups.

The second report on this sample compared therapist-led self-help, partial self-help, and structured self-help in 51 individuals with DSM-IV BED.[327] All three approaches led to significant decreases in objective binges, hours spent bingeing, and body dissatisfaction. Structured self-help led to significantly greater abstinence at the end of treatment but not at followup. Depression scores decreased over time but not differentially across groups. BMI changes did not differ across groups; the authors did not report whether significant decreases occurred within groups, but the numerical changes appeared to be minimal. Dropout was not reported.

Additional interventions for binge eating disorder. In an inpatient trial, Riva et al. compared virtual reality therapy to psychonutritional control in 20 women with DSM IV BED.[330] Virtual reality therapy uses interactive three-dimensional visualization, a head-mounted display, and data gloves to modify body image perceptions. In this very small study with a large number of outcome measures, the investigators compared seven sessions of virtual reality plus a low-calorie diet and physical training with psychonutritional CBT, a low-calorie diet, and physical training. Virtual reality showed significant improvements in weight efficacy and diet scores. Abstinence did not differ significantly between groups and was 100 percent in each, most likely secondary to intensive inpatient treatment. Dropout was not reported.

Summary of behavioral interventions for binge eating disorder. Investigators most frequently chose to study CBT. However, no basic trial comparing individually administered CBT with waiting list, treatment as usual, or a second therapy was rated as fair or good.

The three fair- or good-rated trials that incorporated CBT provided treatment for between 12 weeks and 5 months. Collectively, these trials indicated two main findings. First, CBT is effective in reducing either the number of binge days or the actual number of reported binge episodes. Second, in comparison to waiting list controls, it leads to greater rates of abstinence when administered either individually or in group format, and this abstinence persists for up to 4 months post treatment. CBT also improves the psychological aspects of BED such as ratings of restraint, hunger, and disinhibition. Results are mixed as to whether CBT improves self-rated depression in this population. In all three studies CBT did not lead to decreases in weight. Whether the successful treatment of BED with CBT is associated with less weight gain (as opposed to actual weight loss) over time in individuals with BED has not yet been adequately addressed. Similarly, DBT (one trial) is associated with decreases in binge eating and psychological aspects of the disorder but not with definitive change in depression or anxiety or apparent weight loss.

Although CBT and DBT decrease binge eating and related psychological features of the disorder, they have no observable impact on the important outcome variable of weight loss. This is a somewhat puzzling finding as one would expect decreases in binge eating to be associated with weight loss. The reason for no weight loss is unclear. It is possible that calories previously consumed as binges may be distributed over nonbinge meals; or, how patients label binges and nonbinge meals may change with treatment. In any case, despite reported changes in eating patterns, little demonstrable weight change is achieved.

Self-help (three trials) is efficacious in decreasing binge days, binge eating episodes, and psychological features associated with BED. It also leads to greater abstinence from binge eating when compared to individuals randomized to a waiting list control condition; short-term abstinence rates approximate those seen in face-to-face psychotherapy trials. No self-help trials led to significant decreases in self-rated depression scores or weight in comparison to waiting list controls. Virtual reality therapy must be viewed as experimental; the intensive inpatient treatment associated with this trial invariably affects the perfect abstinence rates observed in both treatment groups. Observing any added efficacy of virtual reality therapy is difficult at best.

Overall dropout rates in behavioral interventions for BED were between 11 percent and 27 percent in active treatment groups.

Key Question 2: Harms of Treatment for Binge Eating Disorder

Table 27 presents adverse events associated with BED treatments. For the trials using second-generation antidepressants, we refer to a recently completed report on the comparative effectiveness and tolerability of second-generation antidepressants (see Chapter 3).[243] In the BED clinical trials, the commonly reported side effects in trials involving fluoxetine were sedation, dry mouth, headache, nausea, insomnia, diarrhea, fatigue, increased urinary frequency, and sexual dysfunction. With fluvoxamine adverse events that occurred significantly more frequently than with placebo included insomnia, nausea, and abnormal dreams. Additional commonly reported adverse events included headache, asthenia, depression, dizziness, somnolence, dry mouth, nervousness, and decreased libido. Patients treated with sertraline experienced insomnia at a significantly greater rate than those receiving placebo; citalopram was associated with more reports of sweating and fatigue than placebo. For tricyclic antidepressants, 24 percent of individuals treated with desipramine discontinued treatment because of side effects. For imipramine, only anticholinergic effects (constipation, dry mouth, blurred vision) were reported more frequently in active drug than placebo participants. In the topiramate trial, six of 30 patients dropped out because of adverse events including headache, parasthesias, and amenorrhea. Individuals treated with sibutramine experienced significantly more constipation than those treated with placebo. Gastrointestinal events were reported more often in individuals receiving orlistat than in those receiving placebo.

No direct adverse events were reported for any psychotherapy trials for BED. In the DBT trial, three individuals required treatment for depression during the follow-up period.

Key Question 3: Factors Associated With Treatment Efficacy

Few studies reported on factors associated with efficacy of treatment in BED. Early abstinence from binge eating was associated with significantly greater weight loss in one study.[316] In one self-help trial, higher initial self-esteem was associated with poorer outcome; however, the effect was small, accounting for 6 percent of the variance in outcome.[326]

Key Question 4: Treatment Efficacy by Subgroups

The total number of individuals enrolled in the 12 drug or medication plus behavioral intervention trials was 680; of those, 55 were men. The age range of participants was reported in eight of the 12 studies; no study reported differential outcome by age. Of the seven studies that did report race or ethnicity, 374 participants were identified as white, 29 as nonwhite, 12 as African American, and six as Hispanic-American. Ten trials were conducted in the United States. No study analyzed results separately by sex, gender, race, or ethnicity. Based on these results, we

Table 27. Adverse events reported: binge eating disorder trials

Intervention	Adverse Events Reported
Medication Trials* †	
Fluoxetine versus placebo[305]	Fluoxetine group: sedation (5), dry mouth (11), headache (9), nausea (7), insomnia (7), diarrhea (6), fatigue (6), increased urinary frequency (4), sexual dysfunction (4). Both groups: hand and foot swelling, palpitations, and apathy; (P = NS)
Fluvoxamine versus placebo[306]	Fluvoxamine group: insomnia, headache, nausea, asthenia, depression, dizziness, somnolence, abnormal dreams, dry mouth, nervousness, and decreased libido. Insomnia, nausea, and abnormal dreams significantly more common in fluvoxamine than placebo.
Fluvoxamine versus placebo[307]	Fluvoxamine group: sedation (8); nausea (4); dry mouth (4); decreased libido (3) Placebo group: sedation (3); nausea (1); dry mouth (3); decreased libido (0) (P = NR)
Sertraline versus placebo[309]	Sertraline group: insomnia (7) Placebo group: insomnia (1) (P = 0.04)
Citalopram versus placebo[308]	Citalopram group: sweating (9) (P = 0.008); fatigue (5) (P = 0.05) Placebo group: sweating (1); fatigue (0) Also reported: dry mouth, headache, diarrhea, nausea, sedation, insomnia, sexual dysfunction
Imipramine versus placebo[310]	Imipramine group: skin eruptions and an aversion to tablet intake (1) anticholinergic effects (7) Placebo group: hunger, sweating, palpitations, arrhythmia, and general malaise (1); anticholinergic effects (3); (P < 0.05)
Topiramate versus placebo[311]	Topiramate group: headache, paresthesias and amenorrhea Placebo: leg cramps, sedation and testicular soreness
Sibutramine hydrochloride versus placebo[312]	Sibutramine: dry mouth (22); headache (6); constipation (7) Placebo: dry mouth (3); headache (14); constipation (0) (P < 0.01) All other adverse events did not differ significantly (i.e., nausea, insomnia, sudoresis, lumbar pain, depressive mood, flu syndrome, malaise, others) (P = NS)
Medication Plus Behavioral Intervention	
Placebo versus fluoxetine versus CBT + placebo versus CBT + fluoxetine[315]	NR
Weight loss treatment versus CBT versus desipramine[316]	8 subjects discontinued desipramine because of side effects
Orlistat plus CBT versus Placebo plus CBT[317]	Orlistat + CBT: significantly more gastrointestinal events
Behavioral Interventions	
Standard CBT versus CBT with spouse involvement versus waiting list control[320]	NR
CBT + exposure versus CBT + cognitive interventions for body image disturbances[319]	NR
CBT versus IPT[318]	NR
Dialectical behavioral therapy versus waiting list control[321]	3 women in DBT group were treated with either psychotherapy or medication for a major depressive episode.

CBT, cognitive behavioral therapy; IPT, interpersonal psychotherapy; NR, not reported; NS, not significant, vs., versus.
* If no numbers appear in parentheses, authors had only listed adverse events but not reported the number of cases.
† P values indicate differences between groups, they are reported when provided by author.

Table 27. Adverse events reported: binge eating disorder trials (continued)

Intervention	Adverse Events Reported
Self-help	
Guided self-help versus pure self-help versus waiting list control[326]	NR
Therapist-led versus partial self-help versus structured self-help versus waiting list control[328]	NR
Therapist-led versus partial self-help versus structured self-help[327]	NR
Other Behavioral Interventions	
Virtual reality based treatment versus psychonutritional control[330]	No adverse events observed

conclude that no information exists about differential efficacy of pharmacotherapy interventions for BED by sex, age, gender, race, ethnicity, or cultural group.

The total number of individuals enrolled in psychotherapy, self-help, or other behavioral trials was 532; of those, 32 were men. Participants ranged in age from 18 to 64. No studies looked at BED treatment for children or adolescents. From the trials that reported race or ethnicity, participants included 450 whites, 19 nonwhites, eight African Americans or Afro-Caribbeans, six Hispanic-Americans, one Native American, and one Asian. In no instance did the investigators analyze results separately by race or ethnic group. No data exist regarding differential efficacy of psychotherapeutic treatment for BED by sex, age, gender, race, ethnicity, or cultural group.

Chapter 6. Outcomes of Eating Disorders

This chapter presents the results of our literature search and findings for key questions (KQs) 5 and 6. KQ 5 asks what factors are associated with outcomes among individuals with the following eating disorders: anorexia nervosa (AN), bulimia nervosa (BN), and binge eating disorder (BED). KQ 6 asks whether outcomes for each of these disorders differ by sex, gender, age, race, ethnicity, or cultural groups.

We report our results separately for each disease in three main sections of this chapter. Use of the term "significant" means that differences over time or between groups were statistically significant at least at the $P < 0.05$ level.

We include literature that discusses more than one disease if findings do not combine individuals with different eating disorders. The review focuses on four main outcomes categories of interest: those related to eating, those involving psychiatric or psychological variables, those measured by biomarkers (e.g., weight, menstruation), and death. Many studies were conducted outside the United States, including Germany, England, Scotland, Sweden, China, Japan, New Zealand, and Australia. For that reason, we note in many cases below the setting (city, country) of the studies to emphasize the extent to which this literature is not directly generalizable to US populations and reflects variations across locales.

We include summary tables containing information on outcomes for studies that we rated fair or good. Similar to text, tables group studies by design: cohort (following a group of individuals, with the disease, identified from the community) or case series (following a group of individuals, with the disease, who received treatment) and whether a nondisease comparison group is followed as well. Articles that discuss results from the same study (the same sample for the same amount of time) are grouped in the same row. Finally, within these categories, we list studies alphabetically by author.

Six of the 62 outcomes articles we identified presenting outcomes for individuals with AN, BN, or BED received a quality rating of "poor;" Table 28 documents the reasons why these studies received this rating. Although each study was not deficient in all areas, common concerns contributing to a low rating included the following: a study involved only participants from one eating disorder program in one location or lacked a description of the location; the study did not have a comparison group; the statistical analysis did not include a power analysis or the authors did not report that they conducted any power analyses; the statistical analysis did not have necessary controls for confounding; and outcome assessors were not blinded to study group or blinding status was not described. As in earlier chapters, we do not discuss these studies further in the text.

For each included study, detailed evidence tables appear in Appendix C.[‡‡] Evidence Table 15 contains the included articles for AN outcomes; Evidence Table 16, articles for BN outcomes; and Evidence Table 17, articles for BED outcomes. Within each table, studies are listed alphabetically. Studies with outcomes for individuals with both AN and BN are in evidence tables for both diseases. To answer KQ 6, we used the literature that met our inclusion criteria and was relevant to answer KQ 5.

[‡‡] Appendixes cited in this report are provided electronically at
http://www.ahrq.gov/downloads/pub/evidence/pdf/eatingdisorders/eatdis.pdf.

Table 28. Outcome studies: reasons for poor quality ratings and number of poor ratings by disease type

Reasons Contributing to Poor Ratings	Types of Disease, Number of Times Flaw Was Detected, and Citations
	Research Aim
Hypothesis not clearly described	Anorexia Nervosa: 0
	Bulimia Nervosa: 0
	Binge Eating Disorder: 0
	Study Population
Characteristics not clearly described	Anorexia Nervosa: 1[331]
	Bulimia Nervosa: 0
	Binge Eating Disorder: 0
No specific inclusion or exclusion criteria	Anorexia Nervosa: 2[331,332]
	Bulimia Nervosa: 1[333]
	Binge Eating Disorder: 0
Study groups not comparable to each other and/or to non-participants with regard to confounding factors or characteristics	Anorexia Nervosa: 0
	Bulimia Nervosa: 0
	Binge Eating Disorder: 0
	Eating Disorder Diagnosis Method
Used independent clinician diagnosis or method used not reported	Anorexia Nervosa: 2[331,334]
	Bulimia Nervosa: 0
	Binge Eating Disorder: 0
None used to diagnose patients similar in treatment/disease and comparison groups	Anorexia Nervosa: 0
	Bulimia Nervosa: 0
	Binge Eating Disorder: 0
	Study Design
Participants drawn from a treatment program in one city or area not reported	Anorexia Nervosa: 5[332,334-337]
	Bulimia Nervosa: 1[333]
	Binge Eating Disorder: 0
No comparison group	Anorexia Nervosa: 6[332,331,334-337]
	Bulimia Nervosa: 1[333]
	Binge Eating Disorder: 0

Table 28. Outcome studies: reasons for poor quality ratings and number of poor ratings by disease type (continued)

Reasons Contributing to Poor Ratings	Types of Disease, Number of Times Flaw Was Detected, and Citations
	Statistical Analysis
Statistics inappropriate	Anorexia Nervosa: 0
	Bulimia Nervosa: 0
	Binge Eating Disorder: 0
No controls for confounding (if needed)	Anorexia Nervosa: 4[331,332,335,336]
	Bulimia Nervosa: 0
	Binge Eating Disorder: 0
Power analysis not done or not reported	Anorexia Nervosa: 5[331,332,334-336]
	Bulimia Nervosa: 1[333]
	Binge Eating Disorder: 0
	Results/Outcome Measurement
Outcome assessor not blinded or not reported	Anorexia Nervosa: 3[331,332,337]
	Bulimia Nervosa: 0
	Binge Eating Disorder: 0
Outcome measures not standard, reliable, or valid in all groups	Anorexia Nervosa: 0
	Bulimia Nervosa: 0
	Binge Eating Disorder: 0
Interpretation of statistical tests inappropriate	Anorexia Nervosa: 0
	Bulimia Nervosa: 0
	Binge Eating Disorder: 0
	External Validity
Population not representative of US population relevant to these treatments	Anorexia Nervosa: 2[331,336]
	Bulimia Nervosa: 0
	Binge Eating Disorder: 0
	Discussion
Results do not support conclusions, taking possible biases and limitations into account	Anorexia Nervosa: 0
	Bulimia Nervosa: 0
	Binge Eating Disorder: 0
Results not discussed within context of prior research	Anorexia Nervosa: 0
	Bulimia Nervosa: 0
	Binge Eating Disorder: 0

Anorexia Nervosa

Our discussion of AN outcomes includes 38 articles exclusively discussing individuals with AN[3,7,177,331,332,334-366] and seven articles discussing individuals with both AN and BN.[367-373] First we discuss results for KQ 5, then KQ 6.

Key Question 5: Factors Associated with Outcomes

Eating-related outcomes. Table 29 presents outcomes from studies rated fair or good; we discuss factors associated with outcomes in the text. Types of studies include prospective cohort with a nondisease comparison group and case series with and without a nondisease comparison group.

Many studies evaluate eating-related outcomes based on the general Morgan-Russell (M-R) scale or some modification of the scale, which evaluates weight (and menstruation in females), or the average M-R scale, which is a composite rating of subscales measuring nutritional status, mental status, sexual adjustment, menstrual functioning, and socioeconomic status. General scale categories are defined as good—normal body weight and regular menstruation—intermediate, amenorrhea *or* low body weight (i.e., weight less than 85 percent of average body weight [ABW]); and poor—amenorrhea *and* low body weight (i.e., less than 85% ABW).

Prospective cohort studies with comparison groups. We included one prospective cohort study with outcomes for individuals with AN in our review that reported results in several articles, after participants were followed for 5 years[345,356] and 10 years.[349,352,362] AN participants were 51 residents of Göteborg, Sweden (including three males), born in 1970, who had been diagnosed with AN as adolescents. Comparisons were Göteborg residents matched to the AN group by age, sex, and school attended. Data from all articles discussing this study did not match exactly; therefore, we caution readers about ostensible trends across time based on data from different studies.

At 5-year followup, approximately one-half of the individuals with AN were considered recovered: 59 percent had no eating disorder (ED) diagnosis and 41 percent had a good outcome according to M-R scale criteria. However, 6 percent still had AN and the remainder had other eating disorders including BN (22 percent) and EDNOS (14 percent). The AN group also remained significantly more symptomatic than the nondisease comparison group on several measures such as dietary restriction, concern about body weight, worry about appearance, and Eating Attitudes Test (EAT) scores.

By 10 years, the M-R scale outcomes had improved. One-half of the cohort who had AN at baseline had a good outcome (49 percent); the percentage of the group with a poor outcome had declined from 24 percent at 5 years to 10 percent at 10 years. Still, 27 percent had an ED diagnosis at followup.

Case series studies with comparison groups. One case series study with a nondisease comparison group discussed results in two articles, Bulik et al.[342] and Sullivan et al.[350] For this study, investigators recontacted 70 women 12 years after referral for treatment (inpatient, outpatient, or assessment) for AN at one facility in Christchurch, New Zealand. The AN group was not limited to those with adolescent onset of the disease. The comparison group (N = 98) resided in the same city and was matched by age. Although 30 percent of individuals with AN at baseline were fully recovered, 21 percent continued to have an eating disorder at followup, with 10 percent continuing to meet Diagnostic and Statistical Manual, version III, Revised

Table 29. Eating-related outcomes: anorexia nervosa

Authors, Year (Quality Score)	Country Sample Size	Outcomes
Prospective Cohort, Comparison Group		
Gillberg et al., 1994[345] (Good)	Sweden	Years followed (mean): 5
Råstam et al., 1995[356] (Good)	Cases: 51 Comparisons: 51	ED dx at FU: AN: 6%; BN: 22%; EDNOS: 14%; None: 59%
		Recovered (M-R scale): 47%
		M-R outcomes: Good: 41%; Intermediate: 35%; Poor: 24%
Nilsson et al., 1999[362] (Good)	Sweden	Years followed (mean): 10
Råstam et al., 2003[349] (Good)	Cases: 51 Comparisons: 51	ED dx at FU: AN: 6%; BN: 4%; EDNOS: 18%; Any ED: 27%
Wentz et al., 2001[352] (Good)		M-R outcomes: Good: 49%; Intermediate: 41%; Poor: 10%
Case Series, Comparison Groups		
Bulik et al., 2000[342] (Good)	New Zealand	Years followed (mean): 12
Sullivan et al., 1998[350] (Good)	Cases: 70 Comparisons: 98	Recovery outcomes: Fully: 30%, Partially: 49%, Chronically ill (current AN, BN or EDNOS): 21%, AN only: 10%
Halmi et al., 1991[7] (Fair)	USA	Years followed (mean): 10
	Cases: 62 Comparisons: 62	ED dx at FU: AN: 3%, BN: 3%, Normal weight bulimia: 23%, EDNOS: 39%, No ED: 27%, Unknown: 5%
Case Series, No Comparison Groups		
Ben-Tovim et al., 2001[367] (Good)	Australia	Years followed (mean): 5
	Cases: 92	ED dx at FU: AN: 21%, BN: 5%, EDNOS: 9%, No ED: 59%, Unknown: 2%, Deceased: 3%
		M-R-H Outcomes: Good: 34%, Intermediate: 54%, Poor: 13%
Dancyger et al., 1997[353] (Fair)	USA	Years followed (mean): 10
	Cases: 52	Recovered: 31%, Good: 13%, Intermediate: 21%, Poor: 35%
Deter et al., 1994[343] (Fair)	Germany	Years followed, mean (range): 11.8 (9-19)
	Cases: 75	Good: 54%; Intermediate: 25% Poor:11%, Deceased: 11%
		AN: 17%
Eckert et al., 1995[338] (Fair)	USA	Years followed, mean (range): 9.6 (8.5 – 10.5)
	Cases: 76	Recovered: 24%, Good: 26%, Intermediate: 32%, Poor: 12%, Deceased: 7%
		ED dx at FU: No ED: 24%, EDNOS: 36%, BN: 22%, AN: 9%, AN/BN: 3%

AN, anorexia nervosa; ANBP, anorexia nervosa binge eating and/or purging subtype; ANR, anorexia nervosa restricting subtype; BED, binge eating disorder; BN,bulimia nervosa; Dx, diagnosis; ED, eating disorder; EDE, Eating Disorder Examination; EDI, Eating Disorder Inventory; EDNOS, eating disorder-not otherwise specified; FU, followup; M-R scores: Morgan and Russell Scale; M-R-H Scale, Morgan-Russell-Hayward Scale; SIAB, Structured Interview for Anorexia and Bulimia Nervosa; Tx, treatment; USA, United States of America.

Table 29. Eating-related outcomes: anorexia nervosa (continued)

Authors, Year (Quality Score)	Country Sample Size	Outcomes
Eddy et al., 2002 (Fair)	USA	Years followed, median (range): 8 (8-12)
	Cases: 136	Full recovery (by subtype): Restricting pure: 46%, Restricting not pure: 22%, Binge/purge:39%
		Relapse from full recovery (by subtype): Restricting pure: 31%, Restricting not pure: 47%, Binge/purge: 68%
		Restricting subtype crossover to binge/purge subtype: 52%
Fichter et al., 1999[339] (Good)	Germany	Years followed (mean): 6.2
	Cases: 95	M-R outcomes: Good: 27%, Intermediate: 25%, Poor: 42% Deceased: 6%
		ED dx at FU: AN: 27%, BN: 17%, EDNOS: 2%, No ED: 55%
Halvorsen et al., 2004[366] (Fair)	Norway	Year followed, mean (range): 8.8 (3.5 – 14.5)
	Cases: 51	M-R outcomes: Good: 80%, Intermediate: 16%, Poor: 4% No ED: 82%, AN: 2%, BN: 2%, EDNOS: 14%
Herzog et al., 1996[370] (Good)	USA	Years followed (mean): 4
	Cases: 76	Full recovery (no symptoms for ≥ 8 wks): ANR: 8%; ANBP: 17% Partial recovery (symptom reduction): ANR: 54%; ANBP: 81%
Herzog, Schellberg et al., 1997[359] (Fair)	Germany	Years followed, mean: 11.7
	Cases:69	Average time to first recovery: 5.8 years
Herzog et al., 1999[369] (Good)	USA	Years followed: Up to 11 (median = 7.5)
	Cases: 136	Full recovery (no symptoms for ≥ 8 wks): ANR: 34%; ANBP: 32% Partial recovery (symptom reduction): ANR: 83%; ANBP: 82% No remission: ANR: 17%; ANBP: 18% Relapse after full recovery: 40%
Isager et al., 1985[340] (Fair)	Denmark	Years followed, mean (range): 12.5 (4 – 22)
	Cases: 142	Average annual hazard rate of relapse: 3%
Lee et al., 2003[347] (Fair) Lee et al., 2005[363] (Fair)	Hong Kong	Years followed: 9
	Cases: 74	M-R scale outcomes: Good: 62% (typical: 52.6%; atypical: 89.47%), Intermediate: 33% (typical: 42.11%; atypical: 5.26%), Poor: 5% (typical: 5.26%, atypical: 5.26%)
		ED dx at FU: No ED: 46% (typical: 40.68%; atypical: 57.14%), AN: 15%, BN: 20% (typical: 25.42%; atypical: 4.76%), EDNOS: 19% (typical: 15.25%; atypical: 28.57%)
Löwe et al., 2001[348] (Fair)	Germany	Years followed (mean): 21.3
	Cases: 63	Full recovery: 51%, Partial recovery: 21%, Poor (including death): 26%, Unknown: 2%
Morgan et al., 1983[355] (Fair)	United Kingdom	Years followed, mean (range): 5.8 (4 – 8.5)
	Cases: 78	M-R Outcomes: Good: 58%, Intermediate: 19%, Poor: 19%, Deceased: 1%, unknown: 3%

114

Table 29. Eating-related outcomes: anorexia nervosa (continued)

Authors, Year (Quality Score)	Country Sample Size	Outcomes
Strober et al., 1997[341] (Fair)	USA	Years followed (range): 10 – 15
	Cases: 93	Full recovery: 76%, Partial recovery: 86%
		Dx of chronically ill at FU: AN restricting: 3%, AN binge eating: 1%, BN: 10%
Tanaka et al., 2001[351] (Fair)	Japan	Years followed, mean (range): 8.3 (4.0 – 17.7)
	Cases: 61	M-R outcomes: Good: 51%, Intermediate: 13%, Poor: 25%, Deceased: 11%

(DSM III-R) criteria for AN. The AN group also continued to exhibit worse eating-related outcomes through other measures. Controlling for age and current AN status, individuals in the AN group reported higher scores on the Eating Disorder Inventory (EDI) drive for thinness and perfectionism subscales and the Three Factor Eating Questionnaire Scale (TFEQ) cognitive restraint and hunger subscales. Similarly, Halmi et al., in a separate US study, found that almost 30 percent of the AN group were recovered at followup.[7]

Case series studies with no comparison groups. Among case series studies with no comparison group, we reviewed three studies limited to patients with adolescent AN onset.[341,366,369,370] Among a mix of 51 former outpatients and inpatients who were followed from 3.5 to 14.5 years in Norway, Halvorsen et al. found that three-quarters of participants no longer had an ED and had a good M-R general scale outcome score.[366] Without controlling for the length of followup, patients who no longer had an ED were significantly less likely to be depressed or suffer from an anxiety disorder, with the exception of obsessive-compulsive disorder, which did not differ across groups.

Similarly, after following 95 patients for 10 to 15 years in the US who had all received inpatient treatment, Strober et al. found that three-quarters of participants had achieved full recovery (free of any symptoms of AN and BN for 8 consecutive weeks).[341] Significant predictors of chronic AN (intermediate or poor outcome) were an extreme compulsive drive to exercise and a history of poor social relating preceding onset of illness. Significant predictors of a longer time to recovery were a more hostile attitude towards one's family and extreme compulsivity in daily routines. In both models, early onset of disease was not a significant predictor.

Using survival analysis, D. Herzog et al. found that a shorter duration of the intake AN episode was a significant predictor of recovery after four years. Other variables in the model that were not significant predictors included age at ED onset, bulimic behaviors, impulse-control behaviors, current depression, and other Axis I disorders.[370] Again, at 7-year followup, the D. Herzog study found a shorter duration of intake episode and higher percentage of ABW at intake predicted both a shorter time to full recovery and a shorter time to partial recovery.[369]

D. Herzog and colleagues compared outcomes for restricting and for binge/purge subtypes of AN. Not all had received inpatient treatment. At up to 4-year followup, the authors found that the percentage of patients who were fully recovered (asymptomatic for at least 8 consecutive weeks) was greater in the AN-binge/purge subtype (17 percent) than in the AN-restricting subtype (8 percent).[370] Corresponding to these descriptive differences, the AN-binge/purge group was

115

significantly more likely to have recovered fully than the AN-restricting group (relative risk [RR], 4.6; 95% confidence interval [CI], 0.98-21.9). A much larger percentage achieved partial recovery (did not meet full criteria for AN but still experienced substantial symptomatology); 81 percent in the binge/purge subtype and 54 percent in the restricting group. At 7-year followup, differences between the groups in the percentage that had recovered had diminished; approximately one-third in both subgroups had fully recovered and more than 80 percent had partially recovered.[369] Forty percent of patients relapsed after first recovery. After following the group for 8 years, differences in duration of disease and ABW predicted being in the binge/purge subtype but measures of impulsivity including a history of alcohol abuse, drug abuse, kleptomania, suicidality, or borderline personality did not.[177]

Through 8-year followup, crossover between the restricting and binge/purge subtypes was high. Of those with the restricting subtype 52 percent changed to the binge/purge subtype, with most of the crossover occurring in the first 5 years of followup.[177] In contrast, Strober et al. found a lower rate of crossover (29 percent); the median time to onset of binge eating was 24 months.[341]

The remaining case series studies discussing eating-related outcomes are not limited to a sample of patients with adolescent onset of AN. First we report outcomes based on M-R scale criteria because they are the most common measures across studies.

A group of females who had all received inpatient treatment in Heidelberg, Germany, were followed up at several points in time. After 6 years, only 27 percent had a good M-R scale outcome, 25 percent had an intermediate outcome, and 42 percent had a poor outcome.[339] However, at later followup points, more than 40 percent of living patients had good outcomes.[338,339,353,354]

Among 74 women, 72 percent of whom had received inpatient treatment for AN, followed for an average of 9 years in Hong Kong, bivariate analyses comparing an M-R outcome of good and Shapiro Control Inventory measures found that a good M-R outcome was associated with a better overall general sense of control, a greater positive sense of control, and a lower negative sense of control.[347,363] A better M-R outcome was also associated with an initial diagnosis of atypical AN (no fat phobia). Using descriptive analyses, Tanaka et al. found, for patients who all had received inpatient treatment, that a good versus poor M-R outcome was associated with younger age at referral, younger age at admission, higher body mass index (BMI) at followup, higher minimum BMI, better menstrual functioning, and better mental state and psychosocial measures.[351]

Morgan and colleagues used bivariate analyses to report on UK patients followed from 4 to 8.5 years, one-half of whom had been hospitalized.[355] They reported that lower general M-R outcome scores were associated with longer duration of food difficulties and longer duration of amenorrhea. Poorer average M-R outcome scores were associated with a longer duration of food difficulties, a longer duration of amenorrhea, greater family hostility towards the patient, a disturbed relationship between the patient and family, and personality difficulties.

Ben-Tovim et al. examined the characteristics of the Morgan-Russell-Hayward Scale (M-R-H scale), a modification of the M-R scale, after adding items related to binge eating and vomiting to a subscale concerning dietary and eating patterns, body concern, and body weight.[367] Using multivariate analyses, the authors found that total M-R-H Scale outcomes were significantly related to the dietary and eating patterns, body concern, and body weight subscale mentioned above. Other subscales measuring menstrual pattern, mental state, psychosexual state, and work and family relations were not significant in the model. Significant predictors in a second model, predicting the same outcome, included subscale 2 at baseline of the disability adjustment scale (measuring overall behavior and social role functioning), the Flinders Medical Centre Symptom Score at baseline (measuring ED symptoms), the Body Attitudes Questionnaire Subscales (measuring a range of body-related attitudes), attractiveness at 6 months, and lastly, change in the salience of weight and shape over the first 6 months of treatment.

Studies also examined diagnostic outcomes, including the persistence of eating disorders over time. Results varied greatly across studies and were not related to length of time to followup. The percentage of individuals who continued to have an AN diagnosis at followup ranged from 9 percent to 29 percent across studies, an EDNOS diagnosis from 2 percent to 36 percent, and no eating disorder from 24 percent to 59 percent of participants.[338,339,363,367,374]

W. Herzog and colleagues measured change over time in the likelihood of first recovery in the Heidelberg case series, after following patients for a mean of 11.7 years.[359] The average patient had a first recovery in 5.8 years, with a greater likelihood of recovering in the first 6 years than later. Significant predictors of first recovery in multivariate models were lower serum creatinine levels at baseline, less purging behavior, and the interaction of less purging and fewer social disturbances as measured by the Anorexia Nervosa Symptom Score (ANSS).

Löwe et al. followed this same group of patients for 21 years.[348] Among the 63 patients, 51 percent showed a good outcome and full recovery, 21 percent were partially recovered, and 26 percent had a poor outcome and 2 percent were unknown. Poor long-term outcome (at 21 years since inpatient admission) was related to low BMI, severe psychological symptoms and social problems, higher EDI perfectionism and interpersonal trust scores, and lower hemoglobin and alkaline phosphatase levels (at 12 years since inpatient admission).

After following this group of patients for 12 years, both Deter and W. Herzog[343] (N = 84, including deceased patients) and Deter et al.[365] (N = 70) found that the persistence of AN symptoms was predicted by older age at onset, more somatic symptoms, more laxative use, low albumin levels, and a high value on a global prognosis score developed from the ANSS.[343,365] Baseline factors associated with relapsing versus having a persistent disorder include being younger, having a shorter disease duration, and less vomiting.[343]

Eckert et al. found, in descriptive analyses in a group of patients who had received inpatient treatment, that recovered patients were less likely to have major affective disorder, anxiety disorders, and phobias.[338]

Isager and colleagues measured relapse rates (lost 15 percent or more of weight gained during course of treatment in a year's time) among 151 patients (93 percent female) who had received treatment (inpatient or outpatient) in Copenhagen, Denmark.[340] After following patients from 4 to 22 years, they found patients were experiencing a 3 percent average annual hazard rate of relapse. Relapse was greater among those whose duration of therapeutic contact was less than 1 year.

Other factors related to these types of outcomes include the following. Factors associated with poor Psychiatric Scale Ratings for AN outcomes in the Fichter and Quadflieg study included binge eating in the month before treatment, other mental illness diagnoses before treatment, and lower body weight at the end of treatment.[339] In research conducted by Lee and colleagues, a group of atypical AN patients scored better at followup on the Eating Attitudes Test – 26 and the Eating Disorders Evaluation Questionnaire.[347,363] Typical versus atypical AN patients at followup had a lower sense of control in the domain of body and a stronger desire for control.

117

Psychiatric/psychological outcomes. Table 30 documents outcomes from eight studies with psychiatric and psychological outcomes.

Prospective cohort studies with comparison groups. The one prospective cohort study that we reviewed followed individuals, at 5 and 10 years, with AN at baseline and compared them with a matched community comparison group in Göteborg, Sweden.[346] At 5 years, the AN group was significantly more likely to have various personality disorders including obsessive-compulsive personality disorder, any Cluster C personality disorder (avoidant, dependent, obsessive-compulsive, or passive aggressive), any personality disorder, or two or more personality disorders as measured by the Structured Clinical Interview II for the DSM-IV (SCID II). In addition, individuals in the AN group had significantly greater rates of Asperger syndrome, any autistic-like condition, and empathy disorder than the comparison group.

At 10 years,[349,352,361,362] the AN group continued to be significantly more likely than the comparison group to currently have a personality disorder, Asperger syndrome disorder or autism spectrum disorder, and lifetime and current obsessive-compulsive disorder. The AN group was not more likely, however, to have an anxiety disorder, excluding obsessive-compulsive disorder.

Ivarsson et al. examined depressive disorders in the AN and comparison groups in these cohorts at both 5- and 10-year followup.[360] The AN group had a higher lifetime prevalence of depression. Being in the AN group was the only significant predictor of depressive disorder at 5-year followup (odds ratio [OR], 7.7; 95% CI, 1.15-19.6). At 10 years, being in the AN group (OR, 4.03; 95% CI, 1.15-14.19) and having a depressive disorder at 5 years were significant predictors of current depressive disorder. The absence of a mood disorder was significantly associated with resolution of the eating disorder.

Case series studies with comparison groups. Two studies followed individuals with AN who had received treatment and a comparison group. Both found higher rates of lifetime major depression and OCD among the AN group.[7,342,350] The study in Christchurch, New Zealand, which followed women for 12 years, found, after controlling for age, significant differences in the lifetime prevalence of several psychological disorders including major depression, mood disorders, obsessive-compulsive disorder, anxiety disorders, and drug dependence.[342,350] The study conducted by Halmi and colleagues also identified that significant differences in the rates of diagnosis of major depression and OCD continued to be true at 10-year followup in their AN case series.[7]

Case series studies with no comparison groups. Descriptively, Eddy et al. found that a history of drug abuse differed among AN subgroups; it was more likely among the binge/purge subtype (16 percent).[177] Correspondingly, among patients who all had adolescent onset of AN, Strober et al., using stepwise regression, found that binge eating at treatment intake was the only significant predictor of the onset of a substance use disorder. Other variables included in the model, such as depression, anxiety, and weight, were not significant predictors.[358]

Also using stepwise regression, Dancyger et al. measured factors related to Minnesota Multiphasic Personality Inventory (MMPI) scores at 10-year followup on a population of women who had received inpatient treatment and were not limited to those with adolescent onset.[353] Poorer overall outcomes were related to higher scores on three MMPI subscales: hypochondriasis, paranoia, and psychopathic deviate.

Table 30. Psychological outcomes: anorexia nervosa

Authors, Year (Quality Score)	Country / Sample Size	Outcomes
		Prospective Cohort Studies, Comparison Groups
Gillberg et al., 1995[346] (Good)	Sweden Cases: 51 Comparisons: 51	Years followed (mean): 5 Diagnoses in AN group*: OCD: 30%, Any cluster C: 37%, any SCID personality disorder: 41%, 2 or more SCID personality disorders: 24%, Asperger syndrome: 12%, any autistic-like condition: 20%; empathy disorder: 30%; OCPD/AS/Autistic-like condition at both age 16 and 21: 45%
Ivarsson et al., 2000[360] (Good) Nilsson et al., 1999[362] (Good) Råstam et al., 2003[349] (Good) Wentz et al., 2000[361] (Good) Wentz et al., 2001[352] (Good)	Sweden Cases: 51 Comparisons: 51	Years followed (mean): 10 Current diagnoses in AN group*: OCD:16%, axis I disorder (including ED): 53% autism spectrum disorder: 18%, cluster C: 22%, Lifetime diagnoses in AN group*: Any affective disorder: 96% OCD: 35%, OCPD:55%, any anxiety disorder: 57%, Any Axis I (including and excluding ED): 100%, depressive disorder: 84%, cluster C: 63%, autism spectrum disorder: 24%
		Case Series, Comparisons Groups
Bulik et al., 2000[342] (Good) Sullivan et al., 1998[350] (Good)	New Zealand Cases: 70 Comparisons: 98	Years followed (mean): 12 Lifetime diagnoses (controlling for age)*: Major depression: Cases: 51%; Comparisons: 36% Any mood disorder: Cases: 60%; Comparisons: 42%, Alcohol or any drug dependence: Cases: 30%; Comparisons: 12% OCD: Cases: 16%; Comparisons: 2% Separation anxiety disorder: Comparisons: 17%; Comparisons: 2% Overanxious disorder: Comparisons: 37%; Comparisons: 3% Any anxiety disorder: Comparisons: 60%; Comparisons: 33%
Halmi et al., 1991[7] (Fair)	USA Cases: 62 Comparisons: 62	Years followed: 10 Lifetime diagnoses*: Major depression: Cases: 68%; Comparisons: 21% Dysthymia: Cases: 32%; Comparisons: 3% Obsessive-compulsive disorder: Cases: 25%; Comparisons: 6% Agoraphobia: Cases: 14%; Comparisons: 3% Social phobia: Cases: 32%; Comparisons: 3% Current diagnoses*: Major depression: Cases: 29%; Comparisons: 6% OCD: Cases: 11%; Comparisons: 2%

*Difference between groups ($P < 0.05$)
AN, anorexia nervosa; AS, Asperger syndrome; CD, compulsive disorder; ED, eating disorder; OCD, obsessive-compulsive disorder; OCPD, obsessive-compulsive personality disorder; sig, significant or significantly; SCID, Structured Clinical Inventory for DSM-IV; USA, United States of America.

Table 30. Psychological outcomes: anorexia nervosa (continued)

Authors, Year (Quality Score)	Country Sample Size	Outcomes
		Case Series, No Comparison Groups
Eddy et al., 2002[177] (Fair)	USA Cases: 246	Years followed (median): 8 History of drug abuse at intake*: AN restricting pure: 0%; AN restricting not pure: 13%; AN binge purge: 16%
Halvorsen et al., 2004[366] (Fair)	Norway Cases: 51	Years followed (mean): 8.8 Diagnosis at followup: Depression: 22%; Anxiety (not OCD): 27%; OCD: 2% Diagnoses at followup*: Depression: No ED group: 13%; ED group: 56% Anxiety disorder (no OCD): No ED group: 20%; ED group: 56%
Löwe et al., 2001[348] (Fair)	Germany Cases: 63	Years followed (mean): 21 Mood disorders by Psychiatric Status Rating Scale outcomes*: Good: 8%; Intermediate: 31%; Poor: 38% Substance use disorders by Psychiatric Status Rating Scale outcomes*: Good: 5%; Intermediate: 6%; Poor: 50%
Strober, Freeman et al., 1996[358] (Good)	USA Cases: 95	Years followed: 10 Substance use disorder: Abuse: 12%; Dependence: 7%

Biomarker-measured outcomes. Table 31 contains study outcomes assessed with biomarkers. This category has very few studies primarily because many studies present measurement of weight and menstrual status through general M-R scale outcomes. These results are included among eating-related outcomes above.

Prospective cohort studies with comparison groups. At 5 years, the study of the Göteborg, Sweden, cohort found that the AN group still weighed significantly less than the non-ED comparison group; more of the AN group was appreciably underweight than the comparison, and while only half of the AN group were near average body weight, nearly all of the comparison group were at that weight.[344,345] Regular or cyclical menstruation was significantly less likely in the AN group, and a large percentage of the AN group had dysdiadochokinesis (an inability to execute rapidly alternating movements).

At 10 years, various measures of weight, including direct measures in kilograms, ABW, and mean BMI (body mass index), did not differ significantly between groups.[349,352,361] However, a significantly larger percentage of the AN group still did not have normal menstrual function and continued to demonstrate dysdiadochokinesis.

Case series studies with comparison groups. The AN cohort in the Christchurch, New Zealand, study had significantly lower BMI than comparison participants when controlling for age and current AN status.[344,345] Desired BMI was also lower in the chronically ill AN group than in recovered individuals or the comparison group.

Case series studies with no comparison groups. Hebebrand et al. examined factors associated with BMI at 0 to 33.6 years followup.[354] A BMI of less than 17.5 at followup (criterion cutoff for AN diagnosis) was related to lower BMI at referral, older age at referral, and younger age at

Table 31. Biomarker outcomes: anorexia nervosa

Authors, Year (Quality Score)	Country Sample Size	Outcomes
Prospective		

Authors, Year (Quality Score)	Country Sample Size	Outcomes
Prospective Cohorts, Comparison Groups		
Gillberg et al., 1994[344] (Good)	Sweden	Years followed (mean): 5
Gillberg et al., 1994[345] (Good)	Cases: 51 Comparisons: 51	Near average body weight at FU*: Cases: 53%; Comparisons: 96% Extremely underweight:* Cases: 8%; Comparisons: 0%
		Regular or cyclical menstruation*: Cases: 50%; Comparisons: 90%
		Dysdiadochokinesis*: Cases: 20%; Comparisons: 2%
Råstam et al., 2003[349] (Good)	Sweden	Years followed (mean): 10
Wentz et al., 2000[361] (Good)	Cases: 51 Comparisons: 51	Mean weight: Cases: 62.3 kg; Comparisons: 63.7 kg
		Regular or cyclical menstruation*: Cases: 65%; Comparisons: 85%
Wentz et al., 2001[352] (Good)		Dysdiadochokinesis*: Cases: 22%; Comparisons: 4%
Case Series, Comparison Group		
Bulik, et al. 2000[342] (Good)	New Zealand	Years followed (mean): 12
Sullivan et al., 1998[342] (Good)	Cases: 70 Comparisons: 98	BMI*: Cases: 20.1 kg/m^2; Comparisons: 25.6 kg/m^2
Case Series, No Comparison Group		
Eckert et al., 1995[338] (Fair)	USA	Years followed (range): 8.5 – 10.5
	Cases: 76	ABW at FU: <85%: 23%; 85%-115%: 73%; >115%: 3% Regular menses: 48%
Löwe et al., 2001[348] (Fair)	Germany	Years followed (mean): 21
	Cases: 63	BMI by Psychiatric Status Rating Scale outcomes*: Good: 21.6; Intermediate: 19.7; Poor: 15.3

*Difference between groups ($P < 0.05$).

ABW, percentage of average body weight; BMI: body mass index; diff, different; FU, Followup; IBW, ideal body weight; kg, kilograms; sig, significant or significantly; USA, United States of America.

followup; by contrast, age at disease onset was not a significant predictor. A higher BMI was also found to be significantly related to a better Psychiatric Status Rating Scale outcome at followup.[348]

Eckert et al. followed patients who had received inpatient treatment 10 years previously.[338] Lower weight was associated with greater food faddishness, laxative abuse, body image disturbance, fear of getting fat, disturbance in sexual adjustment, worse psychological adjustment, disturbed menses, and other weight loss behavior.

Mortality outcomes. Table 32 summarizes results from studies of mortality and risk of suicide in individuals with AN.

Prospective cohort studies with comparison groups. No deaths were reported in the Göteborg, Sweden, study through the 10-year followup.

Case series with no comparison groups. All mortality data were obtained from case series studies without a comparison group. Several studies calculated standardized mortality ratios

Table 32. Mortality outcomes: anorexia nervosa

Authors, Year	Country	
Quality Score	**Sample Size**	**Outcomes**
	**Case Series*, No Comparison Groups**	
Birmingham et al., 2005[3] (Fair)	Canada	Years followed (mean): 7
	Cases: 326	Deaths: N=17 (Suicide: N=7, Pneumonia: N=2, Hypoglycemia: N=2, Liver disease: N=2, Cancer: N=2, Alcohol poisoning: N=1, Subdural hemorrhage: N=1) SMR: 10.5
Crisp et al., 1992[357] (Fair)	England and Scotland	Years followed (mean): 22
	Cases: 168	England: Deaths: N=4 (Anorexia: N=2; Suicide: N=1; Cancer: N=1) (SMR: 1.36 times more likely than women of same age, 1973 – 1989)
		Scotland: Deaths N=8 (Anorexia: N=3; Suicide: N=4; Cancer N=1) (SMR: 4.71 times more likely than women of same age, 1973 – 1979)
Deter et al., 1994[343] (Fair) and Herzog, Schellberg et al., 1997 (Fair)	Germany	Years followed, mean (range): 11.8 (9 – 19)
	Cases: 75 at FU	Deaths: N=9 (AN complications: N=7; Suicide: N=2)
Eckert et al., 1995[338] (Fair)	USA	Years followed, mean (range): 9.6 (8.5 – 10.5)
	Cases: 76	Deaths: N=5 (all complications of AN; no suicides); SMR: 12.8
Eddy et al., 2002[177] (Fair)	USA	Years followed, median (range): 8 (8-12)
	Cases: 136	Deaths by subtype: Restricting pure: 8%; Restricting not pure: 8%, Binge/purge: 6%
		History of suicidality by subtype: Restricting pure: 4%; Restricting not pure: 29%; Binge/purge: 27%
Fichter et al., 1999[339] (Good)	Germany	Years followed (mean): 6.2
	Cases: 95	Deaths: N=6 (Traffic accident during exercise: N=1; Cardiac and renal failure: N=2; Hypocalcemia: N=2; Cardiac failure and cachexia: N=1)
Franko et al., 2004[368] (Good)	USA	Years followed (mean): 8.6
	Cases: 136	Suicide attempts during study period: 22%
Hebebrand et al., 1997[354] (Fair)	Germany	Years followed, mean (range): 9.5, 0 – 33.6
	Cases: 272	Deaths: N=12 (Emaciation: N=10, Suicide: N=2)
		Mortality rate by patient weight at referral: < 13 kg/m^2: 11%, ≥ 13 kg/m^2: 0.6%; BMI < 13 at referral associated with higher likelihood of mortality
Herzog et al., 2000[371] (Fair)	USA	Years followed: 11
	Cases: 110	Deaths: N=7 (Suicide: N=3; Acute alcohol intoxication: N=1; Cardiorespiratory failure, heptic failure, and cirrhosis: N=1; Cardiac arrhythmia and seizure disorder: N=1; Fungal pneumonia: N=1)
		SMR (all deaths): 9.6; SMR (suicide): 58.1

AN, anorexia nervosa; FU, Followup; N, number; sig, significant; SMR, standardized mortality ratio; Tx, treatment; USA, United States of America.

*In case series studies, sample size is as of the date of the analysis and therefore does not include deceased cases.

Table 32. Mortality outcomes: anorexia nervosa (continued)

Authors, Year Quality Score	Country Sample Size	Outcomes
Isager et al., 1985[340] (Fair)	Denmark	Years followed, mean (range): 12.5 (4 – 22)
	Cases: 142	Deaths N=9 (Suicide: N=6, Malnutrition: N= 2, Unknown: N=1)
Keel et al., 2003[372] (Fair)	USA	Years followed (mean): 8.6
	Cases: 136	Deaths: N=11; SMR: 11.6 Suicide: N=4; Suicide SMR: 56.9
Lee et al., 2003[347] (Fair)	Hong Kong	Years followed (mean): 9
	Cases: 80	Deaths: N=3 (Suicide: N=2, Emaciation: N=1); SMR: 10.5
Löwe et al., 2001[348] (Fair)	Germany	Years followed (mean): 21.3
	Cases: 63 at FU	Deaths: N=14 (12 directly due to AN)
Møller-Madsen et al., 1996[364] (Fair)	Denmark	Years followed, mean (range): 7.8 (< 1 – 17)
	Cases: 853	Deaths: N=50 (AN complications: N=13, Natural causes: N=11, Suicide: N=18, Accidents: N=2, Unknown causes or could not be determined: N=4) SMR: Females: 9.2; SMR: Males: 8.2 Females only < 1 year following treatment admission, SMR=30.5
Patton, 1988[373] (Fair)	United Kingdom	Years followed (mean): 7.6 Deaths: N = 11 (Suicide: N = 6; low weight: N = 5)
	Cases: 332	Overall SMR: 6.01; Higher than expected SMR at 4-year FU: 5.76, Higher than expected SMR at 8-year FU: 2.70, Normal level
Sullivan et al., 1998[350] (Good)	New Zealand	Years followed: 12
	Cases: 70	Deaths: N = 1 (suidice)
Tanaka et al., 2001[351] (Fair)	Japan	Years followed, mean (range): 8.3 (4.0 – 17.7)
	Cases: 61 at FU	Deaths: N=7 (Emaciation: N=3; Suicide: N=2; Murder: N=1; Burn: N=1)

(SMR), allowing for comparison to the population based on age, sex, and time when the patient population was drawn.

The SMRs were elevated in the AN groups and ranged from 9 to 13 across studies.[3,338,347,364,371,372] In one study, SMRs were significantly elevated in a female patient population through 14 years of followup (ranging from 30.5 at less than 1 year followup to approximately 6 for the remainder of the period). The SMR was no longer significantly elevated after 14 years.[364]

Only in two studies conducted in the United Kingdom were the SMRs lower. Crisp et al. examined mortality among females more than 20 years after they had received treatment for AN in either London, England (1968 to1973), or Aberdeen, Scotland (1965 to 1973).[357] In England, women with AN were 1.36 times more likely to die than women of the same age in England and Wales between 1973 and 1979. In Scotland, women with AN were 4.71 times more likely to die than women of the same age in Scotland during the same period.

Patton and colleagues conducted a record review of 332 AN patients, mostly female (96 percent), who had received treatment at Royal Free Hospital in the United Kingdom between

1971 and 1981.[373] The SMR at 4-year followup was 5.76, which was a significant elevation; at 8-year followup, the SMR was 2.7 (not significant). Predictors of mortality included weight less than 35 kilograms at presentation and more than one inpatient admission.

In one study that followed patients for 8.6 years, significant predictors of death (controlling for age and duration of illness before intake) included greater severity of alcohol use disorders, greater severity of substance use disorders, worse social adjustment, and worse global assessment of functioning (GAF) scores. Predictors of shorter time to death included longer duration of illness at treatment intake, affective disorder hospitalization at intake, suicidality associated with mental illness other than an ED, substance abuse, and worse severity of alcohol use over the course of the illness.[372] Descriptively, Isager et al. found that deceased patients were significantly more likely to have been hospitalized.[340]

Suicide was a common cause of death. Among the group of females with adolescent AN onset who received ED treatment at the Massachusetts General Hospital or other Boston area clinics the SMR was 58.1, significantly higher than that for the population as a whole.[371]

Franko et al. reported predictors of suicide attempts among the women in the Boston cohort.[368] Thirty percent of their patients had a history of suicide attempts before they entered the study; during the study, 22 percent of AN patients attempted suicide. A history of a suicide attempt at intake significantly predicted time to a future attempt in individuals with AN. Using multiple regression techniques, the authors determined that a first suicide attempt was predicted by a history of suicide attempts at intake, greater drug use, participation in individual therapy, use of neuroleptic medications, and older age at disease onset.

A history of suicidality was significantly different among patient subtypes in one study – lower in the pure restricting group than other groups.[177] However, the groups did not differ in rates of death at 8-year (median) followup.

Several other case series studies that were discussed in relation to their eating, psychological, or biomarker outcomes reported deaths of patients during the followup period. These are summarized in Table 32.

Summary of studies addressing KQ 5. One prospective cohort study following individuals who had AN and a healthy comparison group has been conducted. Limited to individuals with adolescent onset of their illness and comparisons in Göteborg, Sweden, this study found that, over a 10-year period, approximately one-half of the group had fully recovered; a small percentage continued to suffer from AN, and the remainder still had other eating disorders. The AN group no longer differed from the comparison group in terms of weight but these individuals continued to be more depressed than comparisons and to suffer from a variety of personality and obsessive-compulsive disorders, Asperger syndrome, and autism spectrum disorders.

Two case series studies, which gathered followup measures from individuals who had received treatment for AN and a nondisease comparison group, were reviewed. They concluded that individuals with AN continued to be more likely to have eating and comorbid psychiatric diagnoses years after treatment. In one study, lower desired body weight and lower desired and actual BMI continued in the AN group, after controlling for current AN status. Individuals in the AN group were also more likely to be depressed and to suffer from mood and anxiety disorders. The second study, limited to psychiatric outcomes, found continued higher rates of major depression and obsessive-compulsive disorder.

The remaining studies had no comparison groups. Rates of recovery and good outcomes varied across studies. Only a relatively small percentage of patients continued to be diagnosed with AN or BN at long-term followup, but many continued to have eating disorders, and relapse rates were high. We did not find evidence that age of disease onset was related to disease chronicity. A relatively large percentage of patients cross over from the restricting subtype to the binge/purge subtype of the disease, but results are mixed concerning which subtype has better eating outcomes.

Few studies examined psychiatric and psychological comorbidities independently of their relationship to eating disorder outcomes. Among those that did and had a comparison group, individuals with AN had a higher probability of having a depression and anxiety disorders diagnosis (including obsessive-compulsive disorder) than comparison individuals. Based on the results of one cohort study, individuals with AN may also be more likely to have Asperger syndrome or autism spectrum disorder. Among individuals with AN, substance abuse may be associated with binge eating.

Through at least 5 years of followup, individuals with AN are more likely to weigh less than comparisons and evidence suggests that their desired weight is lower. We did not find similar predictors of continued low weight in the AN case series studies and so are unable to draw conclusions concerning these relationships. However, some evidence exists that lower weight at treatment presentation is related to poorer outcomes.

The mortality risk is significantly greater among those diagnosed with AN than in the population as a whole. The risk of suicide is particularly pronounced, as is the risk of death early in the followup period. Increased risk is associated with alcohol and substance use disorders.

Key Question 6: Outcome Difference by Sex, Gender, Age, Race, Ethnicity, or Cultural Group

We examined whether AN outcomes differed by participants' sex, gender, age, race, ethnicity, or cultural groups. We found insufficient evidence to evaluate differences by sex or gender. Males were included in only 19 of 38 reviewed studies and were never more than 10 percent of the analysis sample in any one study. No study included any analyses examining differences controlling for sex or gender.

No study that we reviewed provided outcomes based on the age of the participant at followup. Some studies limited participants to those whose AN onset was during adolescence, but none compared outcomes of those with adolescent onset to those with older onset. However, six studies did include a measure of age at disease onset. Whether this is a significant factor in the course of AN is of particular interest in the field.

Results were mixed. Descriptively, Tanaka et al. found that a good M-R rating was related to younger age at referral;[351] Deter and Herzog found that earlier onset of disease was a significant predictor of AN symptoms at 12-year followup.[343] Suicide attempts were more likely among those whose disease began at an older age.[368] In contrast, Strober et al. did not find age at onset to be a significant factor in predicting chronic AN (intermediate or poor outcomes) at 10- to 15-year followup.[341] It was also not a predictor of time to recovery after 4 years in the Heidelberg case series.[370] Lastly, although Hebebrand et al. found age at onset not to be significantly related to lower BMI at followup,[354] they reported that older age at referral and younger age at followup predicted worse outcome.

Only two studies, both from the United States, reported the race or ethnicity of participants. Nonwhite subjects constituted 4 percent of the Boston, Massachusetts, case series[368] and 7 percent of the case series from the University of California at Los Angeles.[341,358]

Bulimia Nervosa

Our discussion of BN outcomes includes 14 articles exclusively discussing individuals with BN[70,333,375-385] and seven articles discussing individuals with both AN and BN.[367-373] As above for AN, we first discuss results for KQ 5, then results for KQ 6.

Key Question 5: Factors Associated with Outcomes

Eating-related outcomes. Table 33 summarizes results from studies that report eating-related outcomes. The BN literature that met our inclusion criteria included only case series studies (i.e., no cohort studies). One study had a nondisease comparison group; all other studies had no comparison group.

Case series studies with comparison groups. Female patients who had received inpatient treatment (N = 163), in Germany were followed for 12 years.[378] The comparison group (N = 202) included females ages 18 to 30 who had never received treatment for an eating disorder. The Structured Inventory for Anorexic and Bulimic Syndromes, Expert-Rating version (SIAB-EX) was used to compare eating disorder symptoms between cases and comparisons at 12 year followup. The BN group as a whole was significantly more symptomatic than the comparison group, as were individuals with BN who were considered to be recovered.

As shown in Table 33, the BN group improved over time. At 2 years, 53 percent were considered recovered and did not have any ED diagnosis. At 6 years, the same was true of 67 percent of the women and, at 12 years, of 66 percent of the women.[378] However, even though recovery rates improved over time, total EDI scores were worse at 2- and 6-year followup than at discharge.[70]

Lifetime psychiatric comorbidity predicted a significantly higher probability of having any eating disorder at 2- and 6-year followup. This variable was no longer significant at 12 years. In contrast, after 12 years, greater lifetime psychiatric comorbidity significantly predicted a higher probability of having a global eating disorder outcome as measured by the Psychiatric Status Rating Scale (PSR) (OR, 3.71; 95% CI, 1.16-11.91). A lifetime history of AN and older age at disease onset also predicted a worse PSR at 12 years.[378]

Case series studies with no comparison groups. Fairburn and colleagues conducted 5- and 6-year followup assessments of females recruited for two psychotherapy trials in the United Kingdom.[375-377,386] The investigators recruited 102 patients with BN through general practitioners and psychiatrists with no limitations on age at disease onset.

After 5 years, by a variety of measures, the group had improved since baseline and had experienced a significant reduction, in the previous 3 months, in mean objective bulimic episodes, self-induced vomiting episodes, and laxative misuse.[375] Eating Disorder Examination (EDE) interview measures that significantly improved included those measuring restraint, shape concern, weight concern, and eating concerns.

Fairburn et al. examined whether outcomes differed between persistent disease (at least two episodes of behavior at one or both of last two assessments) and remitted disease (not engaged in any relevant behavior over past 3 months); they focused solely on binge eating or compensatory behaviors.[377] The persistence of binge eating behavior was related to baseline duration of disturbed eating, overvaluation of shape and weight, and worse social adjustment. None of the tested baseline factors predicted compensatory behavior. However, binge eating and compensatory behaviors were significant predictors of each other.

Table 33. Eating-related outcomes: bulimia nervosa

Authors, Year (Quality Score)	Country Sample Size	Outcomes
**Case Series, Comparison Groups**		
Fichter and Quadflieg, 2004[378] (Fair)	Germany	Years followed: 12
	Cases: 163	Case diagnosis at 6 year FU: Recovered/no ED: 67%; AN: 4%; BN purge: 21%; BN nonpurging: 1%; BED: 1%; EDNOS: 1%;Deceased: 1%
	Comparisons: 202	Case diagnosis at 12 year FU: Recovered/no ED: 66%; AN: 2%; BN purge: 10%; BN nonpurging: 1%; BED: 2%; EDNOS: 14%; Deceased: 3%
**Case Series, No Comparison Groups**		
Ben-Tovim et al., 2001[367] (Good)	Australia	Years followed: 5
	Cases: 86	Diagnosis at FU: AN: 1%; BN: 8%; EDNOS: 13%; No ED:74%; Unknown: 5%; Deceased: 0
		M-R-H Outcomes: Good: 76%; Intermediate: 19%; Poor: 2%; Unknown: 2%
Fairburn et al., 2000[375] (Good) Fairburn et al., 2003[377] (Good) Stice and Fairburn, 2003[386] (Fair)	United Kingdom	Years followed: 5
	Cases: 92	Diagnosis at FU: BN: 15%; BED: 7%; AN: 1%; EDNOS: 32% Any DSM-IV ED: 49%; Remission: 35%; Relapse: 26%
Fichter and Quadflieg, 1997[70] (Fair)	Germany	Years followed (mean): 6.2
	Cases: 185	Diagnosis at 2 years FU: AN: 2%; BN: 36%; EDNOS: 8%; No ED: 55% Diagnosis at 6 years FU: AN: 4%; BN: 21%; BED: 1%; EDNOS: 2%; No ED: 71%
Herzog et al., 1993[380] (Good)	USA	Years followed: 1
	Cases: 96	First shift to subclinical BN diagnosis (loss of full criteria without considering duration): 86% Partial recovery: 71%; Full recovery: 56%
Herzog et al., 1996[370] (Good)	USA	Years followed: 4
	Cases: 150	Partial recovery: 88%; Full recovery: 57%
Herzog et al., 1999[369] (Good)	USA	Years followed (Median): 7.5
	Cases at baseline: 110	Full recovery: 74%; Partial recovery: 98%; Relapse after full recovery: 35%
Jäger et al., 2004[381] (Fair)	Germany	Years followed: 8
	Cases: 80	Diagnosis at FU: BN: 29%; EDNOS (bulimic): 9%; EDNOS (anorexic): 1%; No ED diagnosis: 61% No binges per week at FU: 63%

AN, anorexia nervosa; BED, binge eating disorder; BN, bulimia nervosa; DSM-IV, Diagnostic and Statistical Manual for Mental Disorders, Fourth Edition; ED, eating disorder; EDNOS, eating disorder not otherwise specified; FU, followup; M-R-H Scale, Morgan-Russell-Hayward Scale; USA, United States of America.

Table 33. Eating related outcomes: bulimia nervosa (continued)

Authors, Year (Quality Score)	Country Sample Size	Outcomes
Keel et al., 1999[384] (Fair)	USA	Years followed (mean): 11.5
Keel, Mitchell, Davis et al., 2000[383] (Fair)	Cases: 173	Diagnosis at FU: BN: 11%; AN:1%; BED: 1%; EDNOS: 19%; lifetime history of AN: 36%; lifetime history of BED: 11%
Keel, Mitchell, Miller et al., 2000[385] (Fair)		Narrow definition of remission: Full: 42%, Partial: 28% Broad definition of remission: Full: 47%, Partial: 23%

At 6-year followup, using multivariate analysis, Fairburn, Norman et al. determined that significant predictors of current AN or BN status (adjusted for the type of treatment received and the duration of followup) included paternal obesity (OR, 5.73; 95% CI, 1.56-21.1) and premorbid obesity (OR, 4.31; 95% CI, 1.35-13.7).[376]

Stice and Fairburn categorized their BN patients into dietary and dietary-depressive subtypes using cluster analysis.[386] Compared with persons in the dietary subtype, those in the dietary-depressive subtype were significantly more likely to have lifetime psychiatric treatment for eating disorders at baseline and during followup, greater persistence of binge eating and compensatory behaviors, and diagnoses of major depression, panic disorder, obsessive-compulsive disorder, social phobia, generalized anxiety disorder, and agoraphobia.

D. Herzog and colleagues examined eating-related outcomes for a group of female patients who sought treatment at Massachusetts General Hospital and other Boston area ED programs.[369,370,380] The authors examined levels and predictors of full and partial recovery at 1, 4, and 7 years. Full recovery was defined as 8 consecutive weeks of being asymptomatic; partial recovery was defined as not meeting full criteria for AN or BN but still experiencing significant symptomatology.

The percentage of the group that fully recovered increased over time. At 1 year, 56 percent were fully recovered;[380] at 4 years, 57 percent were fully recovered;[370] and at 7 years, 73 percent had achieved a full recovery at some point during followup.[369] The trend was similar for partial recovery at some point during followup: 1 year, 71 percent;[380] 4 years, 91 percent;[370] and at 7 years, 98 percent.[369] Recovery was not, however, necessarily persistent even if it covers 8 consecutive weeks. By 7 years, 35 percent had relapsed after achieving a full recovery.

The authors investigated predictors of recovery at each followup. At 1 year, ideal body weight (IBW) was not a significant predictor of time to partial recovery.[380] Variables included in their models at both 4- and 7- year followup included duration of the current disorder episode, age at onset of the current eating disorder, age at onset of the first eating disorder, weight, binge and purge frequency, and the co-occurrence of various other disorders including those involving a lack of impulse control, depression, personality and any Axis I disorder. At both points, no significant predictors of recovery emerged from among these variables.[369,370]

Ben-Tovim et al. analyzed results from 86 female BN patients who had been treated by an eating disorder specialist in Adelaide, South Australia, and followed for 5 years.[367] Not all had inpatient stays and age at onset was not reported. Using multivariate analyses, they reported that total M-R-H scale outcomes were significantly related to subscales for dietary and eating patterns, body concern, and body weight rather than other subscales concerning menstrual pattern, mental state, psychosexual state or work and family relations. In a second multivariate model, M-R-H total scores were predicted by overall behavior and social functioning at baseline, feeling fat at study recruitment, attractiveness at 6 months, and change in depression over the first 6 months.

Jäger et al. compared outcomes of female patients who had received analytic inpatient and systemic outpatient treatment at a hospital in Germany.[381] Over time, binges, bulimia severity, the number of episodes of food restriction, and EAT measures of bulimia and dieting significantly decreased in both treatment groups; in addition, the number of normal meals increased. The group receiving analytic inpatient treatment had a greater decline in the severity index and the number of restrictions than the group receiving systemic outpatient therapy.

Keel and colleagues examined eating-related outcomes for 173 females with a mean of 11.5 years following evaluation at the University of Minnesota's Eating Disorders Clinic.[383-385] Members of the group had participated in one of two previous treatment studies. A particular interest in this study was comparing results based on different definitions of remission. Defining remission as freedom from disordered eating for at least 6 months and the absence of undue influence of shape and weight on self-evaluation, the authors reported that 42 percent were in full remission and 28 percent in partial remission. Using a broader definition of remission, including absence of disordered eating for at least 8 weeks with no restrictions based on the influence of weight and shape, they reported 47 percent were in full remission and 23 percent were in partial remission.[384]

The authors compared the relation between prognostic factors and two specifications of the outcome measure: categorical (full or partial remission vs. not in remission) and continuous (log of the number of months since last binge/purge episode).[384,385] The two models showed little difference in results. Significant factors in relation to both outcome specifications included lifetime substance use, baseline substance use, current mood, substance use, and impulse control disorders, and results on a multidimensional personality questionnaire. Prognostic factors that were not statistically significant in relation to either outcome specification included age at onset, duration of symptoms at baseline, baseline depression or anxiety disorder, and lifetime mood or anxiety disorder.

Keel et al. compared the association among six definitions of BN outcomes and a variety of other outcome measures and prognostic variables.[383] Definitions of BN outcomes varied based on the duration of abstinence required for full remission or recovery, the number of categories in which outcomes were placed, and how the categories were combined. Full recovery ranged from 47 percent to 38 percent based on the required duration of abstinence in the specification. Other outcomes that were significantly related to the eating disorder outcome in all specifications included depression, body image disturbance, impulse control, and social adjustment. The analysis did not identify any prognostic factors that were statistically significant in relation to all six eating disorder specifications. However, substance abuse was significant in four of six specifications, age of presentation in three specifications, and age of onset in two.

Including 101 of the females from the University of Minnesota study discussed above, Keel et al. also examined the independence and relative strength of depression compared with bulimic symptoms in predicting body dissatisfaction at followup.[382] Baseline depression was both independent of and superior to bulimic symptoms in predicting body dissatisfaction at followup, demonstrating a direct association between depression and body dissatisfaction that is independent of bulimic symptoms.

Psychiatric/psychological outcomes. Table 34 summarizes results from studies reporting psychiatric/psychological outcomes.

Table 34. Psychological outcomes: bulimia nervosa

Authors, Year (Quality Score)	Country Sample Size	Outcomes
Case Series, Comparison Groups		
Fichter and Quadflieg, 2004[378] (Fair)	Germany Cases: 163 at 12 year followup Comparisons: 202	Years followed: 12 Psychiatric comorbidity at followup: Lifetime 79.7%; current: 41.1% Mood disorders: Lifetime: 69.0%; current: 16.5% Major depression: Lifetime: 58.2%; current: 10.8% Anxiety: Lifetime: 36.1%; current: 22.2% Substance use: Lifetime 36.1%; current: 14.6% Borderline personality disorder: 9.5%
Case Series, No Comparison Groups		
Fichter and Quadflieg, 1997 (Fair)	Germany Cases: 185	Years followed (mean): 6 Psychiatric comorbidity at 2-year followup: Borderline personality disorder: 5%; Substance abuse: 24%; Mood disorders: 30%; Anxiety disorders: 13% Psychiatric comorbidity at 6-year followup: Borderline personality disorder: 4%; Substance abuse: 21%; Mood disorders: 46%; Anxiety disorders: 32%
Stice and Fairburn, 2003 (Fair)	United Kingdom Cases: 82	Years followed: 5 Psychiatric comorbidity at followup:* Major depression: Dietary: 61%; Dietary-depressive: 81% Panic disorder: Dietary: 15%; Dietary-depressive: 33% Obsessive-compulsive disorder: Dietary: 2%; Dietary-depressive: 25% Generalized anxiety disorder: Dietary: 11%; Dietary-depressive: 47% Agoraphobia: Dietary: 4%; Dietary-depressive: 36%

*Difference between groups ($P < 0.05$).

Prospective cohort studies with comparison groups. The Fichter and Quadflieg study that followed females with BN and a healthy comparison group recorded psychiatric comorbidities in the BN group only.[70,378] In the first 6 years after treatment, general psychopathology, as measured by the Symptom Checklist 90-Revised (SCL-90), found that symptoms were worse at 2-year followup but better at 6-year followup compared to the end of treatment.[70] At 12 years, 80 percent of patients had a lifetime psychiatric disorder, and 41 percent had a psychiatric disorder in the month before assessment. Half of the patients had suffered from a lifetime mood disorder or major depression and 36 percent had suffered from an anxiety or substance use disorder.[378]

Case series studies with no comparison groups. The Jäger et al. study that reported 8-year outcomes following either analytic inpatient or systemic outpatient treatment found that depression had declined in both groups[381] but that the decline was greater in those who received inpatient treatment.

Biomarker measured outcomes. Table 35 presents results from studies with outcomes assessed through various biomarkers.

Case series studies with no comparison groups: Gendall et al. followed 82 females for 1 year who had participated in outpatient treatment trials in New Zealand.[379] At followup, approximately 31 percent of the female participants had irregular menses. In multivariate analyses, irregular menses (irregular or absent menstrual cycles within the past 3 months) were significantly related to a greater maximum-minimum weight difference and current smoking.

Table 35. Biomarker outcomes: bulimia nervosa

Authors, Year (Quality Score)	Country Sample Size	Outcomes
	Case Series, No Comparison Groups	
Fairburn et al., 2000[375] (Good)	England Cases: 92	Years followed: 5 Change over time: Weight: 69.8 kg, BMI: 25.5
Fichter and Quadflieg, 1997 (Fair)	Germany Cases: 185	Years followed (mean): 6 Weight at followup: Good (19<BMI<30): 74%; Intermediate (BMI 30-40 or 17.5-19): 17%; Poor (BMI<17.5 or >40): 9%
Gendall, Bulik et al., 2000[379] (Good)	New Zealand Cases: 82	Years followed: 1 Irregular menses: 30.5%
Keel et al., 1999[384] (Fair)	USA Cases: 173	Years followed (mean): 11.5 BMI: 22.1, Weight: 60.7 kg

BMI, Body mass index, measured in kg/m^2; USA, kg, kilograms; United States of America.

Several studies reported improvements over time in weight measures. After 5 years, Fairburn and colleagues found that participants' mean weight and BMI had increased.[375] At 6-year followup, Fichter and Quadflieg found that 74 percent of their participants were in the good weight range.[70] Similarly, Keel et al. measured differences in weight variables in 173 females followed for approximately 11 years.[384] BMI, actual weight, desired weight, and highest weight all significantly increased over time.

Mortality outcomes. Table 36 gives the results from studies that reported on either death or risk of suicide (or both) among individuals with BN.

Case series studies with comparison groups. In the Fichter and Quadflieg study, 2.5 percent of the BN group were deceased at 12-year followup.[378] The SMR was 2.36, not significantly different from the rate expected in the population matched by age and sex.

Case series studies with no comparison groups. Franko et al. reported predictors of suicide attempts in a group of 110 women with BN who had been recruited because they sought treatment for eating disorders at Massachusetts General Hospital and other Boston area clinics.[368] At baseline, 23 percent reported a history of suicide attempts before assessment, and 11 percent reported suicide attempts during the study. After approximately 9 years of followup, significant predictors of shorter time to first suicide attempt included receiving group therapy, receiving individual therapy, younger age at onset, a history of drug use disorder, paranoid personality disorder at intake, and greater severity of laxative use.

In a companion study, D. Herzog et al. followed this same group of women in Boston for 11 years to examine rates and causes of death.[371] At the end of that time, none of the women were deceased.

Keel et al. measured the mortality rates among 110 females, also recruited in Boston, in the same manner as Herzog et al., but the parameters of the recruitment dates differed somewhat. Participants were followed for a median of 9 years.[372] One individual died during the followup period. The SMR of 1.3 was not significantly different from what would be expected in the population as a whole.

Table 36. Mortality outcomes: bulimia nervosa

Authors, Year Quality Score	Country Sample Size	Outcomes
		Case Series Studies, Comparison Groups*
Fichter and Quadflieg, 2004[378] (Fair)	Germany Cases: 163 at 12 year followup Comparisons: 202	Years followed: 12 BN Cases Deaths: 2 year followup: 0 6 year followup: 2 12 year followup: 4, SMR: 2.36
Franko et al., 2004[368] (Good)	USA Cases: 110	Years followed: 8.6 Suicide attempts: 11% Predictors of time to first suicide attempt (adjusted): Group therapy; Younger age at onset; History of drug use disorder; Individual therapy; Paranoid personality disorder; Greater severity of laxative use
Herzog, et al., 2000[371] (Fair)	USA Cases: 110	Years followed: 11 Loss to followup deaths: 0
Keel et al., 2003[372] (Fair)	USA Cases: 110	Years followed (Median): 9 Deaths: 1, SMR: 1.3
Patton et al. 1988[373] (Fair)	USA Cases: 96	Years followed: 4-15 Deaths: N=3 (2 car accidents, 1 low weight) Crude mortality rate: 3.3, SMR: 9.38

BN, bulimia nervosa; SMR, standardized mortality ratio; USA, United States of America.
*In case series studies, sample size is as of the date of the analysis and therefore does not include deceased cases.

Patton et al. measured mortality rates in patients in the United Kingdom who were followed for 4 to 15 years.[373] Three patients died during the observation period, one from low weight. Again, the SMR was not statistically significant from what would be expected in the healthy population.

Summary of findings. All of the BN literature is case series, that is, studies that follow individuals over time who have received treatment. One study included a nondisease comparison group. Much of the emphasis in the BN literature concerned comparing various definitions of disease outcomes and diagnostic subtypes. Generally in these studies, more than half of the patients followed no longer had a BN diagnosis at the end of the study period. A substantial percentage continued to suffer from other eating disorders, but BN was not associated with an increased mortality risk. A limited number of analyses uncovered factors significantly associated with outcomes of this disease. Only depression was associated with worse outcomes consistently across studies.

Key Question 6: Outcome Difference by Sex, Gender, Age, Race, Ethnicity, or Cultural Group

In each of the BN outcomes studies except for Patton et al., all participants we reviewed were female.[373] Four percent of the participants in the Patton et al. study were male; however, this study included both AN and BN populations, and the authors do not specify how many of the included males were in each disorder group.

Most studies did not report the race, ethnicity, or cultural group of the participants. Franko et al. reported that 4 percent of their sample was nonwhite, but they did not specify the distribution in the BN sample, relative to the AN sample.[368] Johnson and colleagues reported that the modal race was white;[333] Keel and colleagues reported that 1 percent of their sample was nonwhite.[384] These investigators did not, however, report outcome differences by race, ethnicity, or cultural group. No outcome studies of BN controlled for the age of participants at entry; no studies were limited to individuals with adolescent onset of the disorder. We conclude that no evidence exists to determine whether outcomes for BN differ by any of these categories.

Binge Eating Disorder

Given the recent addition of the provisional criteria for BED to the psychiatric nomenclature, three studies met our inclusion criteria for this section. All three studies were case series.[387-389] One study included a comparison group.[389] One study was conducted in the United States (rated as fair),[388] one in Germany (rated as fair),[387] and one in Italy (rated as fair).[389]

Key Question 5: Factors Associated with Outcomes

In KQ 5 we address outcomes of BED and factors associated with outcomes. We partitioned outcomes into eating-related outcomes, psychological outcomes, and biomarker outcomes (largely weight change).

Case series with comparison groups. The only case series with a comparison group explored a special population of individuals undergoing laparoscopic adjustable gastric banding.[389] This is an important research question intended to determine whether individuals with BED who are obese are appropriate for bariatric surgery. In this large study of 130 BED patients versus 249 obese comparison individuals without BED, those with BED experienced more band adjustments and more pouch and esophageal dilatations than those without BED. The authors did not report on psychological outcomes. At 5 years, the groups did not differ on measures of either weight loss or weight regain. The authors did not report on any variations in disordered eating behavior that may have persisted after bariatric surgery.

Case series without comparison groups. Fichter et al.[387] followed 62 cases with BED for 6 years; of these patients, 78 percent had no ED diagnosis, 6 percent continued to have a BED diagnosis, and a minority had developed BN or EDNOS over the followup interval. Over the 6-year interval, depression, anxiety, and obsessionality measures also improved. The authors did not report whether changes observed in BMI over time were significant. No additional factors associated with outcome were reported.

The second case series examined the impact of comorbid psychopathology and personality disorders on treatment outcome for BED.[388] Individuals with cluster B personality disorders reported a greater number of binge days at 1-year followup. Neither binge frequency nor EDE global scores were related to other comorbid conditions. The authors did not report additional psychological or biomarker outcomes.

Summary of studies addressing KQ 5. Only sparse evidence addresses factors associated with BED outcomes. The three included studies have vastly different designs and research questions; more importantly, their findings do not converge.

Key Question 6: Outcome Difference by Sex, Gender, Age, Race, Ethnicity, or Cultural Group

KQ 6 addresses whether outcomes differ for BED by sex, gender, age, race, ethnicity, or cultural groups In all, 405 women and 134 men participated in outcome studies of BED. No study compared differential factors associated with outcome by sex or gender.

Only one study reported ethnicity:[388] 151 whites, five blacks, four Hispanics, and two Native Americans. This study did not report any differential outcomes by ethnicity.

All three studies were of adults. No outcome studies of BED in children have been performed. Nothing is known about differential outcome by age group.

Chapter 7. Discussion

This chapter discusses our findings about anorexia nervosa (AN), bulimia nervosa (BN), and binge eating disorder (BED), which derive from our systematic review of literature for six key questions (KQs). Four KQs dealt with evidence about treatment issues (Chapters 3, 4, and 5):

1. Efficacy of treatments or combination of treatments
2. Harms associated with the treatment or combination of treatments
3. Factors associated with the efficacy of treatment
4. Differences in efficacy of treatment by sex, gender, age, race, ethnicity, or cultural group.

Two other KQs covered the course and outcomes of these conditions (Chapter 6):

5. Factors associated with outcomes among individuals with these conditions
6. Differences in outcomes by sex, gender, age, race, ethnicity, or cultural group.

Our report focused on randomized controlled trials (RCTs) for AN, BN, and BED and on outcomes studies that included sample sizes of 50 or greater and included at least 1 year of follow-up. All studies were published since 1980.

In this chapter, we first review the quality of the literature and the strength of the evidence based on the outcomes of and treatment of eating disorders. The confidence that readers can have in our findings, conclusions, inferences, and research recommendations rests heavily on the quality of the research reviewed and the overall robustness of the evidence. We then discuss the major issues resolved (or not resolved) in treating and managing patients with these conditions, drawing as appropriate from the findings for all six questions. Following that section, we present our research recommendations. The chapter ends with a brief recapitulation of our conclusions.

Critical Findings and Implications for Treatment of Eating Disorders

In this section we review our main findings on treatments for AN, BN, and BED, with specific attention to medications only, behavioral or psychotherapy interventions only, combination approaches, and novel interventions. We also comment on issues relating to outcomes from the disorders, including mortality. Before presenting the findings, we document our approach to assessing the strength of these bodies of evidence. Interpreting our findings accurately requires appreciation of the considerable drawbacks to much of this literature.

Quality of Literature and Strength of Evidence

As described in Chapter 2 and documented in both evidence and summary tables, we first applied rigorous selection criteria for articles and assessed the quality of each study. We then evaluated the strength of the bodies of evidence available to address each KQ for each disorder. The possible grades in our scheme are as follows:

I. Strong evidence. The evidence is from studies of strong design; results are both clinically important and consistent with minor exceptions at most; results are free from serious doubts about generalizability, bias, or flaws in research design. Studies

135

with negative results have sufficiently large samples to have adequate statistical power.

II. Moderately strong evidence. The evidence is from studies of strong design, but some uncertainty remains because of inconsistencies or concern about generalizability, bias, research design flaws, or adequate sample size. Alternatively, the evidence is consistent but derives from studies of weaker design.

III. Weak evidence. The evidence is from a limited number of studies of weaker design. Studies with strong design either have not been done or are inconclusive.

IV. No published literature (for those situations in which no study addressed the question).

For the four treatment KQs, we found the strength of the body of evidence to be of mixed quality that varied considerably across the three disorders (Table 37). For KQ 1, evidence for treatment efficacy, we judged the AN literature to be weak (III); the exception was for psychotherapy for adolescents with AN, for which more evidence was available yielding a moderate rating (II). The strongest treatment efficacy literature was for BN; we judged both medication and behavioral interventions as strong (I), although we gave self-help and other interventions only a weak rating (III). For BED, both medication and behavioral interventions were viewed as moderate (II) with self-help and other interventions as weak (III).

Regarding harms of therapy (KQ 2), we gave strong ratings (I) to the literature on medication interventions for BN and BED. The evidence for harms of other interventions for all three disorders received ratings of either weak (III) or nonexistent (IV). Behavioral trials rarely reported harms associated with treatment.

KQ 3 dealt with factors associated with or influencing therapeutic outcome. With the exception of behavioral interventions for BN, which we rated moderate (II), we rated the literature for all three disorders as weak (III). Very few well-designed studies addressed those factors that lead to good or poor outcome in clinical trials.

Finally, KQ 4 addressed differences in treatment outcome by age, sex, gender, race, ethnicity, or cultural group. For all three disorders and all types of interventions, we rated the

Table 37. Strength of evidence concerning four treatment key questions

Interventions	KQ 1	KQ 2	KQ 3	KQ 4
Anorexia Nervosa				
Medication and Medication plus Behavioral Interventions				
Adults	III	III	III	IV
Adolescents	III	III	III	IV
Behavioral Interventions				
Adults	III	IV	III	IV
Adolescents	II	IV	III	IV
Bulimia Nervosa				
Medication and Medication plus Behavioral Interventions				
All ages	I	I	III	IV
Behavioral Interventions				
All ages	I	IV	II	IV
Self-help				
All ages	III	IV	III	IV
Other				
All ages	III	IV	III	IV
Binge Eating Disorder				
Medication and Medication plus Behavioral Interventions				
Adult	II	I	III	IV
Behavioral Interventions				
Adult	II	IV	III	IV
Self-help				
Adult	III	IV	III	IV
Other				
Adult	III	IV	III	IV

literature as nonexistent (IV). The treatment literature for eating disorders has virtually ignored all these factors.

As reported in Table 38, we found considerable evidence to address factors related to outcomes among individuals with AN and BN (KQ 5) and rated the evidence for both of these disorders as moderate (II). In contrast, the evidence available to address factors related to BED outcomes (KQ 5) was much more limited and, thus, weak (III).

The AN outcomes literature includes one prospective cohort study (following individuals identified in the community) with a comparison group design and one case series study (following a treatment population) with a comparison group design. The remaining literature follows case series of patients without comparisons. Some studies use strong methodological designs that control for length of followup and the effect of independent predictors. However, results were not consistent across studies.

Table 38. Strength of evidence concerning two outcomes key questions

Eating Disorder	KQ 5	KQ 6
Anorexia nervosa	II	III
Bulimia nervosa	II	IV
Binge eating disorder	III	IV

The BN outcomes literature included no prospective cohort studies but did include several studies with strong methodological designs, including one case series study with a comparison group. However, partially because the literature is inconsistent in the methodology used to measure outcome, few factors were found to be consistently related to outcomes and so uncertainty remains.

The BED literature included only three studies. Much of the data provided in these studies was descriptive and offered very limited information concerning factors related to outcomes.

We used the body of literature that met our inclusion criteria for answering KQ 5 to address KQ 6 concerning differences in outcomes by sex, gender, age, race, ethnicity, or cultural group. We graded the AN literature as weak (III) and the BN and BED literature as nonexistent (IV). The AN literature had limited evidence discussing the effect of age of onset on outcomes, but results were not conclusive. The AN literature yielded no evidence to evaluate differences in outcomes by any other KQ 6 criteria. No study addressed any of these concerns for BN and BED.

Our review supports and extends previous systematic reviews on treatment of eating disorders, including several Cochrane reports. Broadly, Cochrane reviews of AN treatment concur that the literature is weak, made no specific recommendations regarding AN treatment, and encouraged larger well-designed trials.[390] For psychotherapy for BN and binge eating, a Cochrane review supported cognitive behavioral therapy (CBT) for BN, in individual or group format, and encouraged further study of self-help.[391] For antidepressant treatment, Cochrane reviewers concluded that single antidepressant agents were clinically effective for BN in comparison to placebo, with greater remission rate but also greater dropouts. No differential effect regarding efficacy and tolerability among the various classes of antidepressants was reported.[392] Examining combinations of psychotherapy and antidepressants for BN, another Cochrane review reported that combination treatments were superior to psychotherapy alone, that psychotherapy appeared to be more acceptable to participants, and that the addition of antidepressants to psychological treatments decreased the acceptability of the psychological intervention.[393]

In addition, guidelines from the National Institute of Clinical Effectiveness (NICE) in the United Kingdom (http://www.nice.org.uk/) concur that AN evidence is weak. The NICE authors assigned high grades to CBT for BN and BED and to antidepressants for BN. For both BN and BED, NICE recommended self-help as an initial treatment step.

Managing Patients with Medication Alone

Managing individuals with AN with medication only is inappropriate, based on evidence reviewed here. No pharmacological intervention for AN has a significant impact on weight gain or the psychological features of AN. Although mood may improve with tricyclic antidepressants, this outcome is not associated with improved weight gain. Moreover, medication treatment for AN is associated with high dropout rates, suggesting that the currently available medications are not acceptable to individuals with AN.

For BN, good evidence indicates that fluoxetine (60 mg/day) reduces core bulimic symptoms of binge eating and purging and associated psychological features of the eating disorder in the short term. Based on two studies, the 60 mg dose performs better than lower doses and may contribute to decreased relapse at 1 year; however, patients do not tend to remain on the drug. Preliminary evidence exists for other second-generation antidepressants (trazodone and fluvoxamine), an anticonvulsant (topiramate), and a tricyclic antidepressant (desipramine). Preliminary evidence exists that monoamine oxidase inhibitors (MAOIs) are associated with decreased vomiting in the treatment of BN, although diet should be closely monitored.

Medication trials for BED have focused primarily on overweight individuals with BED. In these individuals, desired outcomes are twofold: weight loss and abstinence from binge eating. The majority of medication research for BED reflects short-term trials. Preliminary efficacy has been shown for selective serotonin reuptake inhibitors (SSRIs), one serotonin, dopamine, and norepinephrine uptake inhibitor, one tricyclic antidepressant, one anticonvulsant, and one appetite suppressant. In the absence of abstinence data and long-term followup, however, we do not know whether observed changes in binge eating, depression, and weight persist.

Managing Patients with Behavioral Interventions Alone

For adult AN, we have tentative evidence that CBT reduces relapse risk for adults with AN after weight restoration has been accomplished. By contrast, we do not know the extent to which CBT is helpful in the acutely underweight state, as one study found that a manual-based form of nonspecific supportive clinical management was more effective than CBT and interpersonal psychotherapy (IPT) in terms of global outcomes during the acute phase. No replications of these studies exist.

Family therapy as currently practiced has no supportive evidence for adults with AN and a comparatively long duration of illness. Overall, family therapy focusing on parental control of renutrition is efficacious in treating younger patients with AN; these approaches lead to clinically meaningful weight gain and psychological improvement. Although most studies of family therapy compared one variant of family therapy with another, two studies produced results suggesting that family therapy was superior to an individual therapy for adolescent patients with shorter duration of illness.

For BN, evidence for CBT is strong. Although IPT is also as effective, at 1-year followup, based on one study, symptomatic change appears to be more rapid with CBT. This factor decreases the time that patients are exposed to the symptoms of BN. Dialectical behavioral therapy (DBT) and guided imagery both show preliminary promise for BN patients.

For BED, CBT decreases the target symptom of binge eating. It does not, as currently delivered, promote weight loss in overweight patients. DBT may hold promise for BED patients as well.

Managing Patients with Combination Interventions

Although many of the medication trials for AN were conducted within the context of basic clinical management, no study that systematically studied medication plus psychotherapy for AN met our inclusion criteria.

For BN, the combined drug plus behavioral intervention studies provide only preliminary evidence regarding the optimal combination of medication and psychotherapy or self-help. Although some preliminary evidence exists for incremental efficacy with combined treatment, given the variety of designs used and lack of replication, evidence remains weak.

For BED, the combination of CBT plus medication may improve both binge eating and weight loss outcomes. Sufficient trials have not been done to determine definitively which medications are best at producing and maintaining weight loss in this population. Moreover, the optimal duration of medication treatment for abstinence from binge eating and sustained weight loss has not yet been addressed empirically, yet weight-loss effects of medication are generally known to cease when the medication is discontinued.[394]

Managing Patients with Novel Interventions

Across the three disorders, we found evidence of various innovative approaches that seem to hold promise, especially for conditions as complex as these eating disorders. Nonetheless, nothing can be said definitively because the trials were small and inconclusive.

Reducing Mortality

The AN outcomes literature clearly and consistently identified that the risk of death is significantly higher in the AN population than would be expected in the population in general. Life-threatening complications of the disease include not only those directly related to weight loss and other physical problems but also a significantly elevated risk of suicide.

Studies were inconsistent concerning whether deceased patients had been included in the analysis sample at followup. Therefore, factors related to poor outcomes did not always include mortality risk. Several studies identified factors related to death versus all other outcomes. Only by including death with other outcome categories can we determine if factors related to death differ from factors related to other poor outcomes.

Individuals with BN and BED were not identified as being at elevated risk of death.

Methods and Other Deficiencies in Reviewed Studies and Recommendations to Overcome Them

Sample Sizes, Attrition, and Statistical Power

Adequate sample sizes. Especially in AN clinical trials, sample size was often insufficient to draw conclusions regarding differential efficacy across groups. Even when investigators did power calculations, they often did not plan an adequate allowance for attrition. Given this limitation, researchers using designs that contrasted one approach with another most commonly observed no differences across interventions. This result was especially true in trials of behavioral interventions and even more so in those that included a large number of comparison groups.

Accurate power analyses should be conducted before starting any study and presented in the methods section. Larger multisite studies should be conducted as a means of bolstering patient numbers.

Subgroup analyses. Even in the face of small sample sizes, many authors conducted subgroup analyses on outcome variables, often in the absence of *a priori* hypotheses. In these small studies, the ability to discern even large differences between groups is limited, and some findings might arise by chance. Investigators must avail themselves of adequate statistical assistance to ensure against inappropriate analyses of this sort.

Attrition. Loss to followup and dropout from clinical trials is especially problematic in AN studies.[395] Individuals with AN are often in denial, deeply fearful of weight gain (which is the key treatment outcome), and hesitant to take medication. High attrition compromises the integrity of outcome data; differential attrition between treatment intervention groups and comparison (e.g., usual-care or placebo) groups is even more damaging. In light of high attrition, researchers often reported completer analyses rather than intention-to-treat analyses, and the former practice can bias results.

Substantial attention needs to be paid to enhancing motivation for treatment in individuals with AN and to improving retention in clinical trials. Although dropout is somewhat lower in BN and BED studies than in AN studies, investigators should also address these factors in clinical trials for these disorders.

Study Design and Statistical Analysis Issues

In general, the eating disorders literature suffers from insufficient rigor with respect to statistical design and analysis in both the planning and conduct of trials. This leads to both gaps and inaccuracies in reporting and interpreting results. Minimally, these problems call into question the validity of the conclusions that can be drawn from individual studies. More broadly, it limits cross-study comparisons and the systematic accumulation of findings that stand the test of time and replication. Ultimately, these problems will hinder the advancement of effective treatments.

Unclear randomization and allocation concealment. Randomization procedures were not of uniformly high standards in the AN, BN, and BED literatures. Many studies failed to report how investigators achieved randomization (if indeed they did achieve it). In many instances, clinical decisions interfered with the integrity of the randomization procedures. No studies reported procedures for allocation concealment.

Trial design challenges. A common problem involves lack of attention to the within-subject repeated design inherent in intervention and treatment trials. For example, studies often indicate the use of repeated-measures analysis but then actually report analysis of posttreatment outcome data only using a paired *t*-test to identify treatment group differences. In some cases, investigators include baseline data as a covariate (which is not explicitly identical to using a repeated-measures model); in other cases, they do not take baseline data into account at all.

In addition, authors sometimes compute a change (delta) score (posttreatment minus baseline) representing within-subject change over time. This is a reasonable (indeed, often preferable) analytic approach to understand pre-post differences. However, they then fail to account for baseline differences that could result in misinterpretation of mean within-group delta scores; an example is when higher baseline values are associated with smaller delta scores.

Overall, advances in this field demand more clarity in the description of analytical methods employed, including specifically the analytic models that have been determined *a priori*, and for the use of repeated measures models with appropriate inclusion of covariates. Attention to these recommendations should improve our ability to integrate information from disparate studies and to draw conclusions with higher yield with respect to the design and implementation of future interventions.

Duration of treatment and absence of followup. Only a very few studies included a dimension of differential duration of treatment in their designs. Assuming that a medication trial that lasts weeks is likely to have long-lasting effects on symptoms that have been present often for many years is unrealistic. Realistic duration of treatment and longer followup of patients in clinical trials for AN, BN, and BED are essential. In addition, strategies to develop continuation and maintenance treatments have not yet been addressed in this field. They are a critical next step in both medication and psychotherapy research.

Excessive diagnostic and outcome measures. The field of eating disorders has spawned an unusually large array of diagnostic and outcome assessment measures. The lack of consistency of measures renders comparisons across studies virtually impossible. This problem is an especially important barrier to standardizing measures of weight and weight change in outcome assessments and trials involving AN therapies, especially when age and sex corrections for body mass index (BMI) should be employed. Future efforts to refine and consolidate the number of measures would be a valuable contribution to the field.

Researchers should be careful not to include too many outcome measures in their designs. They need to avoid having many outcome variables at the expense of the most important behavioral indicators. Excessive numbers of outcome measures, especially those that may be closely related, lead to a higher likelihood of Type I errors and an inevitable focus on the minor significant findings that do emerge. This is especially detrimental to understanding the efficacy of therapeutic regimens when those findings are not the most clinically relevant dimensions or when their relevance to recovery is unknown.

Treatment of medical morbidities. Insufficient attention has been paid to addressing the optimal approach to treatment of serious long-term physical sequelae of AN and BN, most notably osteoporosis. We advise that measures of physical health issues be considered in the design of future trials.

Sociocultural context. Although the facilitating nature of sociocultural forces such as emphasis on thinness and unhealthy dieting have long been acknowledged, few treatment or outcome studies have attempted to measure the impact of these pernicious contextual factors. Although these variables are less tractable (for study design and conduct) than more readily measured factors such as eating-disordered behaviors, depression, anxiety, or biomarkers, greater attention to developing effective methods to measure these contextual factors may reveal important and often overlooked factors that influence recovery. This in turn may open new avenues for prevention, community education, policy, and strategies for maintenance of treatment gains.

Reporting Issues

Lack of definition of stage of illness, remission, recovery, and relapse. For AN, BN, and BED, investigators did not apply consensus definitions of stage of illness, remission, recovery, and relapse. Developing standardized definitions of these terms for each disorder and the means to evaluate them are high priorities for future research. Accomplishing this will require a concerted and orchestrated effort to bring researchers together to develop such definitions and reporting guidelines.

Reporting change as reduction in behaviors rather than abstinence or remission. Especially in the BN and BED literature, researchers commonly reported outcomes such as percentage reduction in binge days, percentage reduction in binges, or amount of time spent binge eating. Although these are potential indicators of therapeutic change, when used alone they can be misleading because individuals with high weekly binge eating can reduce this behavior by even as much as 50 percent but still be highly symptomatic. Depending on the disorder and core behaviors being targeted, future studies should report either abstinence from binge eating, vomiting, and other compensatory behaviors or absence of binge days for a specified duration of time (at least 1 month but preferably longer).

Statistical reporting. Frequently, authors do not report degrees of freedom, making it impossible to decipher the exact nature of the model being tested. Incomplete reporting of results derived from multivariate models is problematic. Authors should take care to report clearly any interaction, between-group, and within-group effects when they employ repeated designs.

Statistically significant differences versus clinically meaningful differences. Across all three disorders attention to distinguishing between statistically significant and clinically meaningful differences is insufficient. For example, significant differences in weight gain in AN and in weight loss in BED may be observed; however, the extent to which group differences as small as 1 kg to 2 kg truly represent clinically meaningful differences is rarely addressed. Definitions of what constitutes clinically meaningful differences in eating disorders are required.

This issue is even more complex when dealing with psychological features of the eating disorder or associated anxiety or depression. Although significant group differences may emerge in a parameter such as hunger, the extent to which this type of finding reflects improvement in the disorder and is a harbinger for remission remains unknown.

Future Research Needs

Gaps in the Literature for Interventions

Gaps in the literature can be identified for the specific diseases and for broader issues of research across eating disorders. We first examine deficits in the evidence base for the main types of interventions (for one, two, or all three of the conditions), drawing on the points made above about the quality of articles or strength of evidence. We then turn to broader methods and related issues for the entire body of investigations in these conditions.

Medications. Discovering new medications that target the core biological and psychological features of AN, address adverse medical sequelae such as osteoporosis, and enhance motivation and retention in medication trials are critically needed steps. As noted, fluoxetine offers some benefits for BN patients. Additional studies are required to determine the long-term effectiveness of relatively brief medication trials, the optimal duration of medication treatment, and the optimal strategy for maintenance of treatment gains. In addition, work to identify and test novel medications that decrease the urge to purge (e.g., with antiemetics) or reduce the extent to which binge eating and purging are experienced as reinforcing is also warranted. Medication trials should focus on achieving abstinence from binge eating and purging, not merely reducing the frequency with which these behaviors occur. Efforts to improve retention in medication trials for BN are also warranted, as are additional studies combining medications and behavioral interventions.

For BED medication questions, future investigations should take care to report specifically and separately on two outcomes – weight loss and abstinence from binge eating – because weight loss is less applicable to individuals with BED who are of normal weight. Future BED studies should clearly distinguish between normal weight and overweight participants and address whether treatment goals include both cessation of binge eating and weight loss. The impact of high placebo response should be considered in future trials and designs modified accordingly (e.g., sufficiently long placebo run-in phases).

Across all three disorders, no effort has been made to study drug augmentation effects. All trials were monotherapy trials; only a few allowed sequential medication in nonresponders. Investigators should consider augmentation strategies in their future studies.

Behavioral interventions. Strategies for enhancing CBT to change both binge eating and weight loss should be included in the next generation of behavioral studies. They should also focus on strategies for enhancing efficacy of CBT and how best to treat CBT nonresponders. On the basis of preliminary trials, DBT also deserves further study.

Combination interventions. The absence of trials combining medications and behavioral interventions (e.g., psychotherapy) is a serious deficit in the AN literature, and it is striking given that treatment delivered in the community for AN patients is often some form of combination treatment. Future studies must address the efficacy of various combinations of treatments for individuals with AN. Future studies should further explore optimal combinations and how best to combine treatments for BN patients who do not respond to CBT or fluoxetine alone. For BED patients, the needed research centers more on which medications have the greatest efficacy for producing desired outcomes and the optimal duration of medication use.

Novel and "borrowed" interventions. Research on innovative medications and behavioral treatments are warranted, especially given the state of treatment of AN. Medications studied to date have either focused on peripheral symptoms such as depression or anxiety or attempted to capitalize on medication side effects such as weight gain, with the aim of aiding weight restoration in AN. Of special importance will be trials of novel medications that target core biological and cognitive features of the disorders and that are also acceptable to patients.

Similarly, psychotherapies applied to eating disorders have been borrowed from other fields such as depression (CBT and IPT), anxiety disorders (exposure with response prevention), and personality disorders (DBT). We should actively seek to further adapt psychotherapeutic interventions that are tailored to the unique core pathology of eating disorders (e.g., drive for thinness, body dissatisfaction, appetite dysregulation) and that are both efficacious and acceptable to the patients. New behavioral interventions that target motivation to change and encourage retention in treatment are required. Further dismantling of complex therapies such as CBT to determine the active therapeutic components is also warranted.

Other fields are benefiting from the application of new information technologies to the treatment of illness. Adequately powered clinical trials that include the use of email, the Internet, personal digital assistants, text messaging, and other technological advances to enhance treatment will add to future treatment development. These approaches may be well suited to disorders marked by shame, denial, and interpersonal deficits and where availability of specialty care is limited.

Multidisciplinary interventions. Specialist inpatient and partial hospitalization treatment of AN often reflects a multidisciplinary approach: medicine, psychiatry, psychology, nutrition, family therapy, and sometimes additional disciplines such as recreational therapy and occupational therapy. The majority of treatment trials have been monotherapeutic. When they are multidisciplinary, the actual component of multidisciplinarity was rarely a variable on which patients were randomized. Studies that directly address the therapeutic benefits of and optimal approach to multidisciplinary treatment are required.

Maintenance of gains after drug discontinuation. For all three disorders, investigators typically failed to provide adequate follow-up time for medication trials. This means they cannot determine the extent to which positive behavior changes seen during medication administration are maintained over time. At minimum, such studies should have at least 1 year of followup. Especially with BN and BED, for which evidence for the short-term efficacy of medication interventions exists, additional information on maintenance of treatment gains, prevention of relapse, and optimal duration of medication treatment are critical next phases for clinical trials.

Gaps in the Literature for Certain Types of Patients

Patients with anorexia nervosa. AN is a serious psychiatric illness. Treatment research on AN is particularly challenging given the characteristic denial of illness, high drop-out rates from treatment, and the limited population prevalence in any single catchment area. Despite the fact that this is the most challenging eating disorder to treat, our evidence base is scant. Studies tend to be small, inadequately powered, and hence inconclusive. Medications studied to date have either focused on peripheral symptoms such as depression or anxiety or attempted to capitalize on medication side effects such as weight gain, with the aim of aiding weight restoration in AN. Both medication and behavioral intervention trials tend to be derivative—using medications or behavioral interventions that are borrowed from other areas of medicine without focusing on the core symptoms of AN.

We noted above some specific gaps related to medication and psychotherapy interventions. We reiterate here the urgency of more, and better, research on this disease. Trials of novel medications that target the core cognitive symptoms and biological processes of AN and medical sequelae are especially needed to move the field forward.

The literature on AN has failed to distinguish sufficiently between interventions targeted at individuals before or after weight restoration and has failed to address the optimal approach to renutrition. Indeed, whether medication and behavioral interventions have different outcomes depending on weight status remains murky. Given that low weight and malnutrition can interfere with the efficacy of medication and the ability to process information in psychotherapy, the optimal timing of the administration of medications and therapy vis-a-vis weight restoration is a critical question that remains unaddressed.

Patients with eating disorders not otherwise specified (EDNOS). Several treatment centers have reported that the majority of individuals who seek treatment for an eating disorder receive a diagnosis of EDNOS.[88,89] EDNOS is a compound category illustrated in the Diagnostic and Statistical Manual, Version IV (DSM IV), by six examples including BED. Despite the patient characteristics that lead to this diagnosis, investigators appear to have ignored systematically those with EDNOS diagnoses. Given the preponderance of individuals with EDNOS diagnoses in treatment settings, this is a serious shortcoming of the literature.

In part, this gap reflects the greater clarity and homogeneity that investigators can achieve in clinical trials when they recruit only individuals with clearly defined AN or BN. However, the price of this clarity is generalizability and, ultimately, understanding the effectiveness of interventions tested. Although some trials have begun to expand inclusion criteria to reflect typical clinical practice, others have retained strict inclusion criteria. Only by further clarifying clinical syndromes within the current EDNOS category and investigating the optimal approach to treat these conditions will we be able to determine how best to treat the majority of treatment-seeking individuals.

Improved epidemiologic data are required to determine whether the frequency with which EDNOS is seen in the clinic reflects population prevalence rates of the various eating disorders. In addition, active strides should be taken to characterize the syndromes that are captured under the heading of EDNOS and to determine the best way to treat conditions that exist under that umbrella diagnostic category.

The need for additional attention to individuals with EDNOS was clearly shown through our review of the outcomes literature. EDNOS is a common outcome among individuals who formerly had AN or BN. However, virtually nothing is known about the persistence of these conditions.

Age and lifespan orientation. The treatment literatures on AN, BN, and BED differ in how they examine differential therapeutic outcomes by age group. For all three disorders, a more thoughtful lifespan approach is required to determine optimal approaches from childhood through older adulthood.

The AN literature is devoid of medication studies for adolescents; drug trials have focused exclusively on adults. Future medication trials should explore medication efficacy in adolescents and the differential efficacy of medications between adolescents and adults.

In contrast, behavioral interventions have focused more on adolescent patients, possibly because of the existence of various family therapy models that are well suited to the context within which adolescent AN arises. Nonetheless, behavioral interventions should pay greater attention to the appropriateness of various approaches across the lifespan (including duration of illness) and of adaptations that depend on age of the patient.

The extent to which CBT approaches to adolescent treatment of AN were adapted to match the developmental level of the patients is unknown. Likewise, approaches that are effective in adolescents may be inappropriate for adults, although developmentally appropriate adaptations may be worthy of study. For example, the relative efficacy of family therapy for adolescents with AN may signal the important role of the family. However, the family of relevance for an adult with AN may be her or his spouse and children rather than family of origin. Such permutations of the therapeutic approach have not yet been tested.

For BN, most commonly older adolescent and adult patients received the same treatment and researchers made no effort to explore differential outcome by age group. Future studies that delve more into mechanisms of treatment response should take care to explore differential age effects.

For BED, no medication or behavioral intervention trials exist for adolescents. No study enrolled patients younger than 18; many included individuals up to 65 without documenting age effects. The first step for BED research is to acquire epidemiologic data to determine the extent to which this disorder is a problem for adolescents. The second needed step is to explore differential outcomes by age.

Males and females. Although males suffer from eating disorders, they are underrepresented in clinical trials of AN and BN. When included, their numbers are usually too small to be analyzed separately. Clinical trials of BED often include a greater number of men; however, no study has reported on differential efficacy by sex.

This situation can be remedied, first, by better studies comparing the phenomenology of AN, BN, and BED in males and females. Second, more extensive epidemiological data can provide more accurate estimates of the actual sex ratio in the population. Third, efforts should be expanded to explore differential treatment needs and outcomes in males and females across the age spectrum. Fourth, we have no data on whether treatment for eating disorders is best conducted in mixed-sex or single-sex environments. Fifth, multisite trials can be designed to increase sample size of male participants.

We note that much of the literature to date deals with males and females (a construct related to sex and biology). Very little research, apparently, tries to deal with gender (a construct related to socialization and social roles). We believe that more attention to the difference between these ideas, and some effort to understand the impact of gender, and not simply sex, may be valuable in understanding treatment approaches and efficacy.

Race and ethnicity. The majority of the literature on AN fails even to report the race and ethnicity of participants. All descriptions of participants should include this critical parameter. Although the more recent BN and BED literature has improved on this point, no studies of medication or behavioral interventions have addressed the issue of whether treatment efficacy differs by race or ethnic background. This is a serious omission in the literature.

To remedy this shortcoming, we must collect adequate epidemiologic data to provide critically needed information about the frequency with which eating disorders occur across racial and ethnic groups. Such data would provide guidance for planning targeted recruitment in clinical trials and enable researchers to set priorities for approaches to incorporating race and ethnicity into both treatment and outcomes studies. In addition, further exploration of sociocultural factors (e.g., stigma) may also assist with understanding both underdetection and underrepresentation of racial and ethnic minorities in research studies.

Underserved populations. The literature on AN, BN, and BED is devoid of any mention of specific issues of gay, lesbian, transsexual, or transgender individuals. These parameters should be systematically recorded in both treatment and outcome studies.

Gaps in the Overall Evidence Base

The United States' contribution to the literature. The literatures on AN, BN, and BED are geographically imbalanced. Although the United States has contributed considerably to the literature on BN and BED, it has done much less on both the treatment and outcome literature for AN. Although outcome studies of AN may be more difficult in the United States because of the mobility of the population, large-scale multisite treatment trials are perhaps more feasible in the United States given the number of academic treatment centers, the generally shared language, and the size of the population base. The United States should expand its contribution to the global literature for the next phase of treatment studies, especially for AN.

In addition, the unique racial and ethnic composition of the United States could assist with addressing the vacuum of information regarding differential treatment outcome by race and ethnicity across AN, BN, and BED. For the outcomes literature, the majority of literature for AN comes from outside of the United States. The extent to which data from outside the United States accurately reflect outcomes in the United States is unclear.

Replication. The hallmark of good science is replication. One major weakness of the existing literature and a critical need for the future is replication. Once efficacious interventions are identified, adequately powered replication studies should be supported to confirm their effectiveness. Results of such studies would need to be careful to report findings using measures and statistical techniques that would allow for direct comparisons across trials.

Large multisite randomized controlled trials. The majority of eating disorders treatment studies are small, single-site trials. The average sample size of AN trials, 23, illustrates this point robustly. Future multisite trials will facilitate patient recruitment, enhance statistical power, enable meaningful subset analyses, buffer against high drop-out rates, and improve generalizability of results. Working in partnership with insurance companies to enable such trials in the current reimbursement milieu may be critical to success.

Generalizability and key treatment questions in the community. Clinical trials for AN in particular do not adequately reflect the type of treatment typically delivered in the community. Nor do clinical trials for AN address some of the key challenges facing clinicians who treat this disorder in inpatient and partial hospitalization or residential settings.

For low-weight patients with AN, the first treatment challenge is weight restoration. Guidelines from the American Psychiatric Association (APA) suggest that individuals at 75 percent of ideal body weight (IBW) or lower are candidates for inpatient weight restoration, although many other factors influence level of care decisions. When facilities are available, weight restoration occurs in hospital, followed by various levels of step-down marked by increasing autonomy and exposure to real-life eating and emotional situations.

No clinical trials for AN address the optimal approach to inpatient weight restoration that can achieve the most lasting gain. This also includes nutritional trials of optimal approaches to renutrition. No studies address the accuracy of the recommendation for hospitalization at 75 percent IBW. No studies address the optimal conditions under which a patient should be discharged from inpatient treatment and stepped down to less structured environments. Given the financial expense of prolonged inpatient hospitalizations and the toll on both patient and family, the conditions under which extended hospitalizations are superior to intensive outpatient management should be the focus of future studies.

Harms of treatment. Trials of medication or behavioral interventions for patients with AN, BN, and BED do not routinely describe the degree of medical compromise or strategies to monitor for potential harm in malnourished patients. Indeed, behavioral intervention trials often completely overlook the fact that their interventions may have adverse effects on patients. Especially given the high drop-out rates from AN trials, behavioral interventions should pay greater attention to both physical and psychological harms associated with interventions. All studies should report adverse events associated with interventions with these disorders. In addition, with AN, researchers should determine, especially within medication trials, whether adverse events differ between the underweight and the weight-restored state.

Issues in Outcomes Research

Outcomes research and treatment research. One serious gap in the evidence base about eating disorders is the absence of "cross talk" between the outcomes and the treatment literatures. Outcomes literature reveals intriguing problems that persist years after the onset of AN. One example is the presence of autism spectrum disorders reported in the Göteborg cohort.[344-346,349,356] Such observations could provide critical information to individuals designing new interventions for AN. Targeting social information processing deficits, for example, could be one way to enhance AN treatment delivery. Paying greater attention to premorbid traits and traits that persist after recovery or through persistent illness may help to enhance treatment efficacy by identifying new treatment targets.

In addition, greater attention to demographic patterns in outcome studies such as typical age of recovery from AN may assist with better appraising where an individual entering treatment is in the course of her or his illness. This could assist with enhancing engagement in treatment and reducing the number of dropouts.

Prospective cohort studies and comparison groups. Virtually all the outcome results and relationships that we identified came from case series studies. This design limits generalizability beyond the specific treatment population being studied. Only one prospective cohort study has been conducted with individuals identified with AN; none has been done among persons with either BN or BED. Therefore, little evidence exists as to whether outcomes differ across treatment populations, individuals in the general population who suffer from these disorders, and those who may not meet threshold diagnostic criteria yet report symptoms or features of the disorders.

Of particular interest would be studies that address factors associated with successful outcomes in AN or BN; these should explore trajectories of recovery and how current diagnostic nosology captures those trajectories. For example, an individual with AN who is assessed 5 years after the onset of that illness may be given a diagnosis of EDNOS; this pattern fails to acknowledge that the patient is on a *recovery* trajectory from AN. The appropriateness of receiving a diagnostic label (EDNOS) different from the original diagnosis (AN), rather than a specific indicator such as AN in partial remission, has yet to be addressed adequately in the literature.

Tracing outcomes across diagnoses. Many individuals who at one time suffered from AN or BN continue to experience less severe eating disorders in later years. Use of dichotomous or simplistic measures of disease state is increasingly seen as uninformative. Additional research is needed that can sufficiently capture the factors associated with transitions in severity of eating disorder diagnoses.

Statistical methods for outcomes research. Outcomes studies vary in their statistical sophistication. At their best, studies used multivariate techniques to control for the influence of various independent variables on outcomes; they may also employ survival analyses techniques to control for differences in the length of time that patients were followed. At their more rudimentary state, many studies simply presented descriptive comparisons between a series of prognostic factors and outcomes of interest, or they employed techniques more appropriate for exploratory research (e.g., stepwise regression). We encourage investigators doing outcomes research (as contrasted with trials) to plan from the outset on using advanced statistical and analytic methodological approaches.

Impact of weight loss treatment on binge eating. Although not a focus of this review, with the ever-increasing obesity epidemic,[396,397] an important area of study will be the impact of various weight loss treatments on binge eating and on the development of eating disorders and eating-disordered behaviors. Programs developed for obesity prevention and treatment in both children and adults should be carefully monitored to ensure that no untoward effects emerge that increase eating-disordered behaviors.[398-401]

Cost-effectiveness analyses. Only rarely has the cost-effectiveness of interventions for AN, BN, and BED been addressed. At some point, however, some medications, behavioral approaches, or combination therapies will appear to be efficacious in trials or effective in broader trials or observational studies. Then, clinicians, insurers, health plan administrators, and others will want information on the relative cost-effectiveness of different therapeutic options. To provide information to address these questions, future studies should include data collection of costs and cost-effectiveness analyses in their designs.

Conclusions

The literature regarding treatment efficacy and outcomes for AN, BN, and BED is of highly variable quality. For AN, the literature on medications was sparse and inconclusive. No studies combining medication with behavioral interventions met inclusion criteria. Evidence suggests that specific forms of family therapy are efficacious in treating adolescents, and preliminary evidence suggests that CBT may reduce relapse risk for adults after weight restoration and that a manual-based form of nonspecific supportive clinical management may be effective in underweight adults.

For BN, fluoxetine (60 mg/day) decreases the core bulimic symptoms of binge eating and purging and associated psychological features in the short term. CBT administered individually or in groups reduced core behavioral symptoms and psychological features in both the short and long term. How best to treat individuals who do not respond to CBT or fluoxetine remains unknown.

In BED, CBT reduced binge eating and leads to greater rates of abstinence when administered either individually or in group format, persisting for up to 4 months after treatment; however, CBT does not lead to weight loss in individuals with BED. Medications may also play a role in the treatment of BED although further research addressing how best to achieve both abstinence from binge eating and weight loss in overweight patients is required.

Higher levels of depression and compulsivity were associated with poorer outcomes in AN; increased mortality was associated with concurrent alcohol and substance use disorders. Only depression was consistently associated with poorer outcomes in BN; BN was not associated with an increased risk of mortality. Because of sparse data, we could reach no conclusions concerning BED outcomes. We uncovered weak to no evidence to address sociodemographic differences in either treatment or outcomes for any of these disorders.

The quality of the literature about treatment efficacy and outcome for AN, BN, and BED is highly variable. In the treatment literature, the largest deficiency rests with treatment efficacy for AN; we rated this literature as the weakest.

Future AN studies require large numbers of participants, multiple sites, clear delineation of the age of participants, and interventions that are tailored to the unique core pathology and medical sequelae of the illness. For BN, future studies should address novel treatments for the disorder, optimal duration of intervention, and optimal approaches for those who do not respond to medication or CBT. For BED, future studies require better explication of how best to target both binge eating and weight loss goals, optimal duration of intervention, and prevention of relapse.

For all three disorders, exploring additional treatment approaches is warranted. In addition, research teams should pay greater attention to factors influencing outcome, harms associated with treatment, and differential efficacy by age, sex, gender, race, ethnicity, and cultural group. Consensus definitions of remission, recovery, and relapse are essential. For both treatment and outcome literature, greater attention is required to the presentations currently grouped under the heading of EDNOS.

Outcome studies, especially for BN and BED, should emphasize population-based cohort studies with comparison groups and plan for adequate durations of follow-up. Ongoing psychiatric epidemiology studies should routinely include assessments of eating disorders. Epidemiologic studies of BMI and obesity trends should include assessments of eating-disordered behavior. Population-based studies should include measures of disability and impairment associated with eating disorders. For both future treatment and outcome studies, researchers must carefully attend to issues of statistical power, research design, and sophistication and appropriateness of statistical analyses.

References and Included Studies

1. Hoek H, van Hoeken D. Review of the prevalence and incidence of eating disorders. Int J Eat Disord 2003;34:383-96.

2. Sullivan PF. Mortality in anorexia nervosa. Am J Psychiatry 1995;152:1073-4.

3. Birmingham C, Su J, Hlynsky J, et al. The mortality rate from anorexia nervosa. Int J Eat Disord 2005;38:143-6.

4. Watson TL, Andersen AE. A critical examination of the amenorrhea and weight criteria for diagnosing anorexia nervosa. Acta Psychiatr Scand 2003;108(3):175-82.

5. Gendall K, Joyce P, Carter F, et al. The psychobiology and diagnostic significance of amenorrhea in anorexia nervosa. Fertility Sterility In Press.

6. Wonderlich S, Lilenfeld L, Riso L, et al. Personality and anorexia nervosa. Int J Eat Disord 2005;37(Suppl):568-71.

7. Halmi K, Eckert E, Marchi P, et al. Comorbidity of psychiatric diagnoses in anorexia nervosa. Arch Gen Psychiatry 1991;48:712-8.

8. Walters EE, Kendler KS. Anorexia nervosa and anorexic-like syndromes in a population-based female twin sample. Am J Psychiatry 1995;152:64-71.

9. Bulik C, Sullivan P, Fear J, et al. Eating disorders and antecedent anxiety disorders: A controlled study. Acta Psychiatr Scand 1997;96:101-7.

10. Kaye W, Bulik C, Thornton L, et al. Comorbidity of anxiety disorders with anorexia and bulimia nervosa. Am J Psychiatry 2004;161:2215-21.

11. Sullivan PF, Bulik CM, Fear JL, et al. Outcome of anorexia nervosa. Am J Psychiatry 1998;155:939-46.

12. Russell G. Anorexia nervosa and bulimia nervosa. In: Russell G, Hersov L, editors. Handbook of psychiatry 4: the neuroses and personality disorders. Cambridge: Cambridge University Press;1983.

13. Feighner J, Robins E, Guze S, et al. Diagnostic criteria for use in psychiatric research. Arch Gen Psychiatry 1972;26:57-63.

14. American Psychiatric Association. Diagnostic and statistical manual of mental disorders. Third Edition. 3rd edition. Washington, DC: American Psychiatric Association Press; 1980.

15. American Psychiatric Association. Diagnostic and statistical manual of mental disorders. Edition III-R. 3rd, revised edition. Washington, DC: American Psychiatric Association Press; 1987.

16. American Psychiatric Association. Diagnostic and statistical manual of mental disorders. Fourth Edition. Washington, D.C.: American Psychiatric Association Press; 1994.

17. WHO. International statistical classification of diseases and related health problems, tenth revision. Geneva: World Health Organization; 1992.

18. McKnight Investigators. Risk factors for the onset of eating disorders in adolescent girls: results of the McKnight longitudinal risk factor study. Am J Psychiatry 2003;160:248-54.

19. Wittchen HU, Nelson CB, Lachner G. Prevalence of mental disorders and psychosocial impairments in adolescents and young adults. Psychol Med 1998;28(1):109-26.

20. Eagles J, Johnston M, Hunter D, et al. Increasing incidence of anorexia nervosa in the female population of northeast Scotland. Am J Psychiatry 1995;152:1266-71.

21. Jones D, Fox M, Babigan H, et al. Epidemiology of anorexia nervosa in Monroe County, New York: 1960-76. Psychosom Medicine 1980;42:551-8.

22. Lucas AR, Beard CM, O'Fallon WM, et al. Anorexia nervosa in Rochester, Minnesota: A 45-year study. Mayo Clin Proc 1988;63:433-42.

23. Møller-Madsen S, Nystrup J. Incidence of anorexia nervosa in Denmark. Acta Psychiatr Scand 1992;86:187-200.

24. Szmukler G. The epidemiology of anorexia nervosa and bulimia. J Psychiat Res 1985;19:143-53.

25. Willi J, Grossman S. Epidemiology of anorexia nervosa in a defined region of Switzerland. Am J Psychiatry 1983;140:564-7.

26. Milos G, Spindler A, Schnyder U, et al. Incidence of severe anorexia nervosa in Switzerland: 40 years of development. Int J Eat Disord 2004;36:118-9.

27. Hall A, Hay P. Eating disorder patient referrals from a population region 1977-1986. Psychol Med 1991;21:697-701.

28. Hoek H, Bartelds A, Bosveld J, et al. Impact of urbanization on detection rates of eating disorders. Am J Psychiatry 1995;152:1272-8.

29. Joergensen J. The epidemiology of eating disorders in Fyn County Denmark, 1977-1986. Acta Psychiatr Scand 1992;85:30-4.

30. Nielsen S. The epidemiology of anorexia nervosa in Denmark from 1973-1987: a nationwide register study of psychiatric admission. Acta Psychiatr Scand 1990;81:507-14.

31. Willi J, Giacometti G, Limacher B. Update on the epidemiology of anorexia nervosa in a defined region of Switzerland. Am J Psychiatry 1990;147(11):1514-7.

32. Lucas AR, Beard CM, O'Fallon WM, et al. 50-year trends in the incidence of anorexia nervosa in Rochester, Minn.: a population-based study. Am J Psychiatry 1991;148:917-22.

33. Gowers S, Crisp A, Joughin N, et al. Premenarcheal anorexia nervosa. J Child Psychol Psychiatry 1991;32:515-24.

34. Inagaki T, Horiguchi J, Tsubouchi K, et al. Late onset anorexia nervosa: two case reports. Int J Psychiatry Med 2002;32:91-5.

35. Beck D, Casper R, Andersen A. Truly late onset of eating disorders: a study of 11 cases averaging 60 years of age at presentation. Int J Eat Disord 1996;20(4):389-95.

36. Jacobi C, Hayward C, de Zwaan M, et al. Coming to terms with risk factors for eating disorders: application of risk terminology and suggestions for a general taxonomy. Psychol Bull 2004;130:19-65.

37. Walsh B, Bulik C, Fairburn C *et al*. Defining eating disorders. Evans D, Foa E, Gur R *et al*. Treating and preventing adolescent mental health disorders: What we know and what we don't know. New York: Oxford University Press, The Annenberg Foundation Trust at Sunnylands, and the Annenberg Public Policy Center of the University of Pennsylvania;2005.

38. Cnattingius S, Hultman C, Dahl M, et al. Very preterm birth, birth trauma, and the risk of anorexia nervosa among girls. Arch Gen Psychiatry 1999;56:634-8.

39. Lilenfeld L, Kaye W, Greeno C, et al. A controlled family study of restricting anorexia and bulimia nervosa: comorbidity in probands and disorders in first-degree relatives. Arch Gen Psychiatry 1998;55:603-10.

40. Wade TD, Bulik CM, Neale M, et al. Anorexia nervosa and major depression: shared genetic and environmental risk factors. Am J Psychiatry 2000;157(3):469-71.

41. Klump KL, Miller KB, Keel PK, et al. Genetic and environmental influences on anorexia nervosa syndromes in a population-based twin sample. Psychol Med 2001;31(4):737-40.

42. Kortegaard LS, Hoerder K, Joergensen J, et al. A preliminary population-based twin study of self-reported eating disorder. Psychol Med 2001;31(2):361-5.

43. Devlin B, Bacanu S, Klump K, et al. Linkage analysis of anorexia nervosa incorporating behavioral covariates. Hum Mol Genet 2002;11(6):689-96.

44. Grice DE, Halmi KA, Fichter MM, et al. Evidence for a susceptibility gene for anorexia nervosa on chromosome 1. Am J Hum Genet 2002;70(3):787-92.

45. Bergen AW, van den Bree MBM, Yeager M, et al. Candidate genes for anorexia nervosa in the 1p33-36 linkage region: serotonin 1D and delta opioid receptor loci exhibit significant association to anorexia nervosa. Mol Psychiatry 2003;8:397-406.

46. Slof-Op 't Landt M, van Furth E, Meulenbelt I, et al. Eating Disorders: From Twin Studies to Candidate Genes and Beyond. Twin Res Hum Genet 16:467-82.

47. Kaye W, Frank G, Bailer U, et al. Neurobiology of anorexia nervosa: clinical implications of alterations of the function of serotonin and other neuronal systems. Int J Eat Disord 2005;37:S15-9.

48. Barbarich N, Kaye W, Jimerson D. Neurotransmitter and imaging studies in anorexia nervosa: new targets for treatment. Curr Drug Targets CNS Neurol Disord 2003;2:61-72.

49. Kaplan A. Medical aspects of anorexia nervosa and bulimia nervosa. Kennedy SH. Handbook of eating disorders. Toronto: University of Toronto;1993:22-9.

50. Katzman DK. Medical complications in adolescents with anorexia nervosa: a review of the literature. Int J Eat Disord 2005;37 Suppl:S52-9; discussion S87-9.

51. Sharp C, Freeman C. The medical complications of anorexia nervosa. Br J Psychiatry 1993;162:452-62.

52. Bulik C. Eating disorders in adolescents and young adults. Child Adolesc Psychiatr Clin N Am 2002;11(2):201-18.

53. Harris EC, Barraclough B. Excess mortality of mental disorder. Br J Psychiatry 1998;173:11-53.

54. Bulik C, Sullivan P, Fear J, et al. Fertility and reproduction in women with anorexia nervosa: a controlled study. J Clin Psychiatry 1999;2:130-5.

55. Rigotti NA, Neer RM, Skates SJ, et al. The clinical course of osteoporosis in anorexia nervosa. A longitudinal study of cortical bone mass. J Am Med Assoc 1991;265(9):1133-8.

56. Szmukler GI, Brown SW, Parsons V, et al. Premature loss of bone in chronic anorexia nervosa. Br Med J (Clin Res Ed) 1985;290(6461):26-7.

57. Gendall K, Bulik C. The long term biological consequences of anorexia nervosa. Current Nutrition and Food Science in press.

58. American Psychiatric Association Work Group on Eating Disorders. Practice guideline for the treatment of patients with eating disorders (revision). Am J Psychiatry 2000;157(1 Suppl):1-39.

59. NICE. http://www.nice.org.uk/page.aspx?o=101239. National Institute for Clinical Excellence; 2004.

60. Golden N, Katzman D, Kreipe R, et al. Eating disorders in adolescents: position paper of the Society for Adolescent Medicine. J Adolesc Health 2003;33:496-503.

61. American Academy of Pediatrics. Identifying and treating eating disorders. Pediatrics 2003;111:204-11.

62. Beumont P, Hay P, Beumont D, et al. Royal Australian and New Zealand clinical practice guidelines for the treatment of anorexia nervosa. Aust N Z J Psychiatry 2004;38(9):659-70.

63. Striegel-Moore RH, Leslie D, Petrill SA, et al. One-year use and cost of inpatient and outpatient services among female and male patients with an eating disorder: evidence from a national database of health insurance claims. Int J Eat Disord 2000;27(4):381-9.

64. McKenzie JM, Joyce PR. Hospitalization for anorexia nervosa. Int J Eat Disord 1992;11:235-41.

65. Matthias R. Care provision for patients with eating disorders in Europe: What patients get treatment where? Eur Eat Disord Rev 2005;13:159-68.

66. Agras W, Brandt H, Bulik C, et al. Report of the National Institutes of Health Workshop on Overcoming Barriers to Treatment Research in Anorexia Nervosa. Int J Eat Disord 2004;35: 509-21.

67. Anderson C, Bulik C. Gender differences in compensatory behaviors, weight and shape salience, and drive for thinness. Eating Behaviors 2003.

68. Lewinsohn P, Seeley J, Moerk K, et al. Gender differences in eating disorder symptoms in young adults. Int J Eat Disord 2002;32:426-40.

69. Woodside DB, Garfinkel PE, Lin E, et al. Comparisons of men with full or partial eating disorders, men without eating disorders, and women with eating disorders in the community. Am J Psychiatry 2001;158(4):570-4.

70. Fichter MM, Quadflieg N. Six-year course of bulimia nervosa. Int J Eat Disord 1997;22(4):361-84.

71. Braun DL, Sunday SR, Halmi KA. Psychiatric comorbidity in patients with eating disorders. Psychol Med 1994;24:859-67.

72. Brewerton T, Lydiard R, Herzog D, et al. Comorbidity of Axis I psychiatric disorders in bulimia nervosa. J Clin Psychiatry 1995;56:77-80.

73. Bulik C, Sullivan P, Joyce P, et al. Lifetime comorbidity of alcohol dependence in women with bulimia nervosa. Addict Behav 1997;22:437-46.

74. Bushnell JA, Wells E, McKenzie JM, et al. Bulimia comorbidity in the general population and in the clinic. Psychol Med 1994;24:605-11.

75. Herzog DB, Keller MB, Sacks NR, et al. Psychiatric comorbidity in treatment-seeking anorexics and bulimics. J Am Acad Child Adolesc Psychiatry 1992;31(5):810-8.

76. Perez M, Joiner TJ, Lewinsohn P. Is major depressive disorder or dysthymia more strongly associated with bulimia nervosa? Int J Eat Disord 2004;36:55-61.

77. Bulik C, Klump K, Thornton L, et al. Alcohol use disorder comorbidity in eating disorders: a multicenter study. J Clin Psychiatry 2004;65:1000-6.

78. Bulik C, Sullivan P, Carter F, et al. Temperament, character, and personality disorder in bulimia nervosa. J Nerv Ment Dis 1995;183:593-8.

79. Fassino S, Amianto F, Gramaglia C, et al. Temperament and character in eating disorders: ten years of studies. Eat Weight Disord 2004;9:81-90.

80. Steiger H, Gauvin L, Israël M, et al. Serotonin function, personality-trait variations, and childhood abuse in women with bulimia-spectrum eating disorders. J Clin Psychiatry 2004;65:830-7.

81. Bulik C, Sullivan P, Kendler K. Heritability of binge-eating and broadly defined bulimia nervosa. Biol Psychiatry 1998;44(12):1210-8.

82. Wade T, Neale MC, Lake RIE, et al. A genetic analysis of the eating and attitudes associated with bulimia nervosa: Dealing with the problem of ascertainment. Behav Gen 1999;29:1-10.

83. Bulik CM, Devlin B, Bacanu SA, et al. Significant linkage on chromosome 10p in families with bulimia nervosa. Am J Hum Genet 2003;72(1):200-7.

84. Frank G, Bailer U, Henry S, et al. Neuroimaging studies in eating disorders. CNS Spectr 2004;9:539-48.

85. Walsh B, Devlin M. Eating disorders: progress and problems. Science 1998;280:1387-90.

86. Mitchell J, Specker S, De Zwaan M. Comorbidity and medical complications of bulimia nervosa. J Clin Psychiatry 1991;52:13-20.

87. Lasater L, Mehler P. Medical complications of bulimia nervosa. Eat Behav 2001;2:279-92.

88. Fairburn C, Walsh B. Atypical eating disorders (eating disorders not otherwise specified). Fairburn C, Brownell K. Eating disorders and obesity: a comprehensive handbook. 2nd edition. New York: Guilford Press;2002:171-7.

89. Turner H, Bryant-Waugh R. Eating disorders not otherwise specified (EDNOS): profiles of clients presenting at a community eating disorders service. Eur Eat Disord Rev 2003;12:18-26.

90. Stunkard AJ. Eating patterns and obesity. Psychiat Quarterly 1959;33:284-95.

91. Walsh B. Diagnostic criteria for eating disorders in DSM-IV: Work in progress. Int J Eat Disord 1992;11:301-4.

92. Spitzer RL, Yanovski S, Wadden T, et al. Binge eating disorders: its further validation in a multisite study. Int J Eat Disord 1993;13(2):137-53.

93. Spitzer RL, Stunkard A, Yanovski S, et al. Binge eating disorder should be included in DSM- IV: A reply to Fairburn et al.'s " The classification of recurrent overeating: the binge eating disorder proposal". Int J Eat Disord 1993;13(2):161-9.

94. Fairburn CG, Welch SL, Hay PJ. The classifaction of recurrent overeating: The "binge eating disorder" proposal. Int J Eat Disord 1993;13(2):155-9.

95. Garfinkel P, Lin E, Goering P, et al. Bulimia nervosa in a Canadian community sample: prevalence and comparison of subgroups. Am J Psychiatry 1995;152:1052-8.

96. Sullivan PF, Bulik CM, Kendler KS. The epidemiology and classification of bulimia nervosa. Psychol Med 1998;28:599-610.

97. Hay P. The epidemiology of eating disorder behaviors: An Australian community-based survey. Int J Eat Disord 1998;23:371-82.

98. Basdevant A, Pouillon M, Lahlou N, et al. Prevalence of binge eating disorder in different populations of french women. Int J Eat Disord 1995;18:309-15.

99. Spitzer RL, Devlin M, Walsh TB, et al. Binge eating disorder: A multisite field trail of the diagnostic criteria. Int J Eat Disord 1992;11(3):191-203.

100. Bruce B, Agras WS. Binge eating in females: A population-based investigation. Int J Eat Disord 1992;12(4):365-73.

101. Bruce B, Wilfley D. Binge eating among the overweight population: a serious and prevalent problem. J Am Diet Assoc 1996;96(1):58-61.

102. Yanovski S, Nelson J, Dubbert B, et al. Association of binge eating disorder and psychiatric comorbidity in obese subjects. Am J Psychiatry 1993;150:1472-9.

103. Langer L, Warheit G, Zimmerman R. Epidemiological study of problem eating behaviors and related attitudes in the general population. Addict Behav 1992;16:167-73.

104. Warheit G, Langer L, Zimmerman R, et al. Prevalence of bulimic behaviors and bulimia among a sample of the general population. Am J Epidemiol 1993;137:569-76.

105. Bulik C, Sullivan P, Kendler K. Medical and psychiatric morbidity in obese women with and without binge eating. Int J Eat Disord 2002;32:72-8.

106. Fairburn CG, Doll HA, Welch SL, et al. Risk factors for binge eating disorder: a community-based, case-control study. Arch Gen Psychiatry 1998;55(5):425-32.

107. Hudson J, Lalonde J, Pindyck L, et al. Familial aggregation of binge-eating disorder. Arch Gen Psychiatry in press.

108. Reichborn-Kjennerud T, Bulik C, Tambs K, et al. Genetic and environmental influences on binge eating in the absence of compensatory behaviors: a population-based twin study. Int J Eat Disord 2004;36:307-14.

109. Branson R, Potoczna N, Kral J, et al. Binge eating as a major phenotype of melanocortin 4 receptor gene mutations. N Engl J Med 2003;348:1096-103.

110. Hebebrand J, Geller F, Dempfle A, et al. Binge-eating episodes are not characteristic of carriers of melanocortin-4 receptor gene mutations. Mol Psychiatry 2004;9:796-800.

111. Brody ML, Walsh BT, Devlin MJ. Binge eating disorder: reliability and validity of a new diagnostic category. J Consult Clin Psychol 1994; 62(2):381-6.

112. de Zwaan M, Mitchell J, Seim H, et al. Eating related and general psychopathology in obese females with binge-eating disorder. Int J Eat Disord 1994;15:43-52.

113. Wilson G. Relation of dieting and voluntary weight loss to psychological functioning and binge-eating. Ann Intern Med 1993;119:727-30.

114. Marcus MD, Wing RR, Hopkins J. Obese binge eaters: affect, cognitions and response to behavioral weight control. J Consult Clin Psychol 1988;56:433-9.

115. Mussell M, Mitchell J, de Zwaan M, et al. Clinical characteristics associated with binge eating in obese females: a descriptive study. Int J Obes Rel Metab Disord 1996;20:324-31.

116. Fichter MM, Quadflieg N, Brandl B. Recurrent overeating: an empirical comparison of binge eating disorder, bulimia nervosa, and obesity. Int J Eat Disord 1993;14(1):1-16.

117. de Zwaan M, Nutzinger D, Schoenbeck G. Binge eating in overweight women. Comprehen Psychiatry 1992;33:256-61.

118. Wonderlich SA, de Zwaan M, Mitchell JE, et al. Psychological and dietary treatments of binge eating disorder: conceptual implications. Int J Eat Disord 2003;34 Suppl:S58-73.

119. Carter W, Hudson J, Lalonde J, et al. Pharmacologic treatment of binge eating disorder. Int J Eat Disord 2003;34 :S74-88.

120. Lask B, Bryant-Waugh. Anorexia Nervosa and Related Eating Disorders in Children and Adolescence. Hove, East Sussex, UK: Psychology Press; 2000.

121. Hansen RA, Gartlehner G, Lohr KN, et al. Efficacy and safety of second-generation antidepressants in the treatment of major depressive disorder. Ann Intern Med 2005;143(6):415-26.

122. West SL, King V, Carey TS et al. Systems to Rate the Strength of Scientific Evidence. Evidence Report, Technology Assessment No. 47. Rockville, Md.: Agency for Healthcare Research and Quality. AHRQ Publication No. 02-E016;2002.

123. Greer N, Mosser G, Logan G, et al. A practical approach to evidence grading. Joint Commision J Qual Improv 2000;26:700-12.

124. Vandereycken W. Neuroleptics in the short-term treatment of anorexia nervosa. A double-blind placebo-controlled study with sulpiride. Br J Psychiatry 1984;144:288-92.

125. Slade P, Russell G. Awareness of body dimensions in anorexia nervosa: cross-sectional and longitudinal studies. Psychol Med 1973;3(2):188-99.

126. Deter H, Herzog W. The anorexia nervosa symptom score: a multidimensional tool for evaluating the course of anorexia nervosa. in: W. Herzog, Deter HC, Vandereycken W, eds. The Course of Eating Disorders: Long-term Follow-Up Studies of Anorexia and Bulimia Nervosa. New York: Springer;1992:40-52.

127. Parloff M, Kelman HC, Frank JD. Comfort, effectiveness, and self-awareness as criteria for improvement in psychotherapy. Am J Psychiatry 1954; 3:343-51.

128. Probst M, Vandereycken W, Van Coppenolle H, et al. Body size estimation in eating disorder patients: testing the video distortion method on a life-size screen. Behav Res Ther 1995;33(8):985-90.

129. Beck A, Ward C, Mendelson M, et al. An inventory for measuring depression. Arch Gen Psychiatry 1961;4:561-71.

130. Spitzer RL, Yanovski SZ, Marcus MD. Binge Eating Clinical Interview. Pittsburgh: HaPI Record; 1994.

131. Gormally J, Black S, Datson S, et al. The assessment of binge eating severity among obese persons. Addict Behav 1982;7:47-55.

132. Rosen JC, Srebnik D, Salzberg E, Wendt S. Development of a body image avoidance questionnaire. Psychol Assess 1991; 3:32-7.

133. Henderson M, Freeman CP. Bulimic Investigation Test Edinburgh. Br J Psychiatry 1987; 150:18-24.

134. Derogatis L, Melisaratos N. The brief symptom inventory: an introductory report. Psychol Med 1983;13(3):595-605.

135. Cooper P, Taylor M, Copper Z, et al. The development and validation of the Body Shape Questionnaire. Int J Eat Disord 1987;6:485-94.

136. Dowson J, Henderson L. The validity of a short version of the Body Shape Questionnaire. Psychiatry Res 2001;102(3):263-71.

137. Slade P, Dewey ME, Newton T, Brodie D, Gundi K. The development and preliminary validation of the body satisfaction scale. Psychol Health 1990; 4:213-20.

138. Franko D, Zuroff D, Rosenthal F. Construct validation of the Bulimic Thoughts Questionnaire. Society of Behavioral Medicine. 1986.

139. Achenbach T. Manual for the Child Behavior Checklist/4-18 and 1991 Profile. Burlington, VT: University of Vermont, Department of Psychiatry; 1991.

140. Crown S, Crisp AH. Manual of the Crown-Crisp Experiential Index. London: Hodder and Stoughton; 1979.

141. Kovacs M. The Children's Depression Inventory. Psychopharmacol Bull 1985; 21:995-8.

142. Thompson M, Gray JJ. Development and validation of a new body-image assessment scale. J Personality Assess 1995;64(2):258-69.

143. Guy W. Assessment Manual for Psychopharmacology - Revised (DHEW Publ No ADM 76-338). 1976.

144. Welner Z, Reich W, Herjanic B, Jung K, Amado H. Reliability, validity, parent-child agreement studies of the diagnosis interview for children and adolescents (DICA). J Am Acad Child Adolesc Psychiatry 1987; 26:694-53.

145. Schlundt D, Zimering R. The Dieter's Inventory of Eating Temptations: A measure of weight control competence. Add Behav 1988; 13(2):151-64.

146. Johnson C. Initial consultation for patients with bulimia and anorexia nevosa. Garner D, Garfinkel PE. Handbook of Psychotherapy for Anorexia and Bulimia. New York: Guilford Press;1997:19-51.

147. Garner D, Olmsted M, Bohr Y, et al. The eating attitudes test: psychometric features and clinical correlates. Psychol Med 1982;12(4):871-8.

148. Cooper Z, Cooper PJ, Fairburn CG. The validity of the eating disorder examination and its subscales. Br J Psychiatry 1989;154:807-12.

149. Garner D, Olmsted MP, Polivy J. Development and validation of a multidimensional eating disorder inventory for anorexia nervosa and bulimia. Int J Eat Disord 1983;2:15-34.

150. Garner D. Eating Disorder Inventory-2: Professional Manual. Odessa, FL: Psychological Assessment Resources, Inc; 1991.

151. Olson D, Sprenkle D, Russel C. Circumplex model of marital and family systems I: Cohesion and adaptability dimensions, family types and clinical applications. Fam Process 1979; 18:3-28.

152. Skinner H, Steinhauer P, Santa-Barbara J. Family Assessment Measure - III Manual. Toronto Canada: Multi Health System, 1995.

153. Moos RH, MoosBS. Family Environment Scale Manual. Palo Alto, CA: Consulting Psychological Press; 1994.

154. Frost R, Marten PA, Lahart C, et al. The dimensions of perfectionism. Cognitive Therapy and Research 1990;14:449-68.

155. Watson D, Friend R. Measure of socio-evaluative anxiety. J Consult Clin Psychol 1969; 33:448-57.

156. Watson D, Friend R. Measurement of social evaluative anxiety. J Consult Clin Psychol 1969; 33:448-57.

157. Leary M. A brief version of the Fear of Negative Evaluation Scale. Personality Soc Psychol 1983; 9:371-6.

158. Stunkard A, Sørensen T, Schlusinger F. Use of the Danish Adoption Register for the study of obesity and thinness. Res Publ Assoc Res Mental Dis 1983; 60:115-20.

159. Goldberg S, Halmi K, Eckert E, et al. Pretreatment predictors of outcome in anorexia nervosa. J Psychiatry Res 1980;15:239-51.

160. Hamilton M. The assessment of anxiety states by rating. Br J Med Psychol 1959; 32:50-5.

161. Hamilton M. A rating scale for depression. J Neurol Neurosurg Psychiatry 1960; 23:56-62.

162. Shor R, Orne EC. The Harvard Group Scale of Hypnotic Susceptibility, Form A. Palo Alto, California: Consulting Psychological Press; 1962.

163. Luborsky. Principles of psychoanalytic psychotherapy. New York: Basic Books; 1984.

164. Robin A, Foster S. Negotiating parent adolescent conflict: A behavioral family systems approach. New York: Guilford Press; 1989.

165. Horowitz L, Rosenberg SE, Baer BA, Ureno G, Vilasenor VS. Inventory of Interpersonal Problems: Psychometric properties and clinical applications. J Consult Clin Psychol 1988; 56:885-92.

166. Craig A, Franklin J, Andrews G. A scale to measure locus of control of behaviour. Br J Med Psychol 1984;57:173-80.

167. Keller M, Lavori PW, Friedman B, et al. The longitudinal follow-up evaluation. Arch Gen Psychiatry 1987;44:540-8.

168. Millon. Millon Clinical Multiaxial Inventory manual. 3rd edition. Minneapolis, MN: Interpretive Scoring Systems; 1983.

169. Dahlstrom W, Welsh GS, Dahlstrom LE. An MMPI Handbook, Vol. 1 Clinical Interpretation. Rev. edition. Minneapolis, MN: University of Minnesota Press; 1972.

170. Hodgson R, Rachman SJ. Obsessional-compulsive complaints. Behav Res Therapy 1977; 15:389-95.

171. Morgan HG, Russell GF. Value of family background and clinical features as predictors of long-term outcome in anorexia nervosa: four-year follow-up study of 41 patients. 1975. 1975:355-71.

172. Morgan H, Hayward AE. Clinical assessment of anorexia nervosa: the Morgan-Russell outcome assessment schedule. Br J Psychiatry 1988; 152:367-71.

173. Vandenberg S, Kuse A. Mental rotation, a group test of three-dimensional spatial ability. Percept Mot Skills 1978;47:509-604.

174. Robin A, Koepke T, Moye A. Multidimensional assessment of parent-adolescent relations. Psychol Assess 1990; 10:451-9.

175. Dupuy H. The Psychological General Well-Being (PGWB) Index. Wenger N, Mattson ME, Furberg CD, Elinson J, eds. Assessment of quality of life in clinical trials of cardiovascular therapies. New York: Le Jacq;1984:170-83.

176. Wing J, Cooper JE, Startorius N. The measurement and classification of psychiatric symptoms. Cambridge University Press; 1974.

177. Eddy K, Keel P, Dorer D, et al. Longitudinal comparison of anorexia nervosa subtypes. Int J Eat Disord 2002;31(2):191-201.

178. Yanovski S. Binge eating disorder: Current knowledge and future directions. Obes Res 1993;1:306-24.

179. Rathus S. A 30-item schedule for assessing assertive behavior. Behav Therap 1973; 4:398-406.

180. Rosenberg M. Society and the Adolescent Self-Image. Princeton, NJ: University Press; 1965.

181. Endicott J, Spitzer RL. A diagnostic interview: the schedule for affective disorders and schizophrenia. Arch Gen Psychiatry 1978;35:837-44.

182. Stanton A, Garcia M, Green S. Development and validation of the situation appetite measures. Add Behav 1990; 15(5):461-72.

183. Weissman M, Bothwell S. Assessment of social adjustment by patient self-report. Arch Gen Psychiatry 1976; 33:1111-5.

184. Kinston W, Loader P. Eliciting whole-family interaction and a standardized clinical interview. J Fam Ther 1984; 6:347-63.

185. Shapiro DJ, Potkin SG, Jin Y, Brown B, Carreon D, Wu J. Measuring the psychological construct of control. Discriminant, divergent, and incremental validity of the Shapiro Control Inventory and Rotter's and Wallstons' Locus of Control Scales. Int J Psychosom 1993; 40(1-4):35-46.

186. First M, Spitzer RL, Gibbon M, Williams JBW. The structured clinical interview for DSM-IV Axis I Disorders. New York: State Psychiatric Institute, Biometrics Research Department; 1994.

187. Zung W. A self-rating depression scale. Arch Gen Psychiatry 1965;12:63-70.

188. Ware J, Snow K, Kosinski M, Gandek B. SF-36 Health Survey: Manual and Interpretation Guide. 1993.

189. Fichter M, Elton M, Engel K, et al. Structured interview for anorexia and bulimia nervosa (SIAB): development of a new instrument for the assessment of eating disorders. Int J Eat Disord 1991;10:571-92.

190. Angold A, Costello E, Messer S, et al. The development of a short questionnaire for use in epidemiological studies of depression in children and adolescents. Int J Meth Psychiat Res 1995;5:237-49.

191. McConnaughy E, Prochaska J, Velicer W. Stages of change in psychotherapy: Measurement and sample profiles. Psychother: Theory Res Pract 1983;20(3):368-75.

192. Rosenthal N, Bradt TH, Wehr TA. Seasonal Pattern Assessment Questionnaire. Washington DC: National Institute of Mental Health; 1987.

193. Spielberger C, Gorsuch R, Lushene R. Manual for the state-trait anxiety inventory. Palo Alto, CA: Consulting Psychologists Press; 1970.

194. Spielberger C. State-Trait Anger Expression Inventory. Tampa, FL: Psychological Assessment Resources, Inc., 1988.

195. Wolpe J. Psychotherapy by reciprocal inhibition. Stanford, CA: Stanford University Press; 1958.

196. Bagby M, Parker J, Taylor G. The twenty-item Toronto Alexithymia Scale - I. Item selection and cross-validation of the factor structure. J Psychosom Res 1994;38:23-32.

197. Cloninger C, Svrakic DM, Przybeck TR. A psychobiological model of temperament and character. Arch Gen Psychiatry 1993;50(12):975-90.

198. Stunkard A, Messick S. The three-factor eating questionnaire to measure dietary restraint, disinhibition and hunger. J Psychosom Res 1985; 29:71-83.

199. Wechsler D. Manual for the Wechsler Adult Intelligence Scale (WAIS). New York: Psychological Corporation, 1955.

200. Clark M, Abrams D, Niaura RS. Self-efficacy in weight management. J Consult Clin Psychol 1991;59:739.

201. Boath E, Pryce A, Cox J. Social adjustment in childbearing women: the modified Work Leisure and Family Life Questionnaire. J Reproduct Infant Psychol 1995;13(3-4):211-8.

202. Sunday S, Halmi KA, Einhorn A. The Yale-Brown-Cornell Eating Disorder Scale: A new scale to assess eating disorders symptomatology. Int J Eat Disord 1995; 18(3):237-45.

203. McElroy SL, Arnold LM, Shapira NA, et al. Topirmate in the treatment of binge eating disorder associated with obesity: a randomized placebo-controlled trial. Am J Psychiatry 2003;160(2):255-61.

204. Goodman W, Price L, Rasmussen S, et al. The Yale-Brown Obsessive Compulsive Scale (Y-BOCS). Arch Gen Psychiatry 1989;46:1006-11.

205. Achenbach T. Manual for the young adult self report and young adult behavior checklist. Burlington, VT: University of Vermont; 1997.

206. Attia E, Haiman C, Walsh BT, et al. Does fluoxetine augment the inpatient treatment of anorexia nervosa? Am J Psychiatry 1998;155(4):548-51.

207. Kaye WH, Nagata T, Weltzin TE, et al. Double-blind placebo-controlled administration of fluoxetine in restricting- and restricting-purging-type anorexia nervosa. Biol Psychiatry 2001;49(7):644-52.

208. Halmi KA, Eckert E, LaDu TJ, et al. Anorexia nervosa. Treatment efficacy of cyproheptadine and amitriptyline. Arch Gen Psychiatry 1986;43(2):177-81.

209. Biederman J, Herzog DB, Rivinus TM, et al. Amitriptyline in the treatment of anorexia nervosa: a double-blind, placebo-controlled study. J Clin Psychopharmacol 1985;5(1):10-6.

210. Klibanski A, Biller BM, Schoenfeld DA, et al. The effects of estrogen administration on trabecular bone loss in young women with anorexia nervosa. J Clin Endocrinol Metab 1995;80(3):898-904.

211. Miller KK, Grieco KA, Klibanski A. Testosterone administration in women with anorexia nervosa. J Clin Endocrinol Metab 2005;90(3):1428-33.

212. Hill K, Bucuvalas J, McClain C, et al. Pilot study of growth hormone administration during the refeeding of malnourished anorexia nervosa patients. J Child Adolesc Psychopharmacol 2000;10(1):3-8.

213. Birmingham CL, Goldner EM, Bakan R. Controlled trial of zinc supplementation in anorexia nervosa. Int J Eat Disord 1994;15(3):251-5.

214. Barbarich NC, McConaha CW, Halmi KA, et al. Use of nutritional supplements to increase the efficacy of fluoxetine in the treatment of anorexia nervosa. Int J Eat Disord 2004;35(1):10-5.

215. Ruggiero GM, Laini V, Mauri MC, et al. A single blind comparison of amisulpride, fluoxetine and clomipramine in the treatment of restricting anorectics. Prog Neuropsychopharmacol Biol Psychiatry 2001;25(5):1049-59.

216. Brambilla F, Draisci A, Peirone A, et al. Combined cognitive-behavioral, psychopharmacological and nutritional therapy in eating disorders. 2. Anorexia nervosa--binge-eating/purging type. Neuropsychobiology 1995;32(2):64-7.

217. Fassino S, Leombruni P, Daga G, et al. Efficacy of citalopram in anorexia nervosa: a pilot study. Eur Neuropsychopharmacol 2002;12(5):453-9.

218. Szmukler GI, Young GP, Miller G, et al. A controlled trial of cisapride in anorexia nervosa. Int J Eat Disord 1995;17(4):347-57.

219. Ricca V, Mannucci E, Paionni A, et al. Venlafaxine versus fluoxetine in the treatment of atypical anorectic outpatients: a preliminary study. Eat Weight Disord 1999;4(1):10-4.

220. Birmingham CL, Gutierrez E, Jonat L, et al. Randomized controlled trial of warming in anorexia nervosa. Int J Eat Disord 2004;35(2):234-8.

221. Eisler I, Dare C, Hodes M, et al. Family therapy for adolescent anorexia nervosa: the results of a controlled comparison of two family interventions. J Child Psychol Psychiatry 2000;41(6):727-36.

222. Lock J, Agras WS, Bryson S, et al. A comparison of short- and long-term family therapy for adolescent anorexia nervosa. J Am Acad Child Adolesc Psychiatry 2005;44(7):632-9.

223. Pike KM, Walsh BT, Vitousek K, et al. Cognitive behavior therapy in the posthospitalization treatment of anorexia nervosa. Am J Psychiatry 2003;160(11):2046-9.

224. McIntosh VV, Jordan J, Carter FA, et al. Three psychotherapies for anorexia nervosa: a randomized, controlled trial. Am J Psychiatry 2005;162(4):741-7.

225. Channon S, de Silva P, Hemsley D, et al. A controlled trial of cognitive-behavioural and behavioural treatment of anorexia nervosa. Behav Res Ther 1989;27(5):529-35.

226. Treasure J, Todd G, Brolly M, et al. A pilot study of a randomised trial of cognitive analytical therapy vs educational behavioral therapy for adult anorexia nervosa. Behav Res Ther 1995;33(4):363-7.

227. Crisp AH, Norton K, Gowers S, et al. A controlled study of the effect of therapies aimed at adolescent and family psychopathology in anorexia nervosa. Br J Psychiatry 1991;159:325-33.

228. Dare C, Eisler I, Russell G, et al. Psychological therapies for adults with anorexia nervosa: randomised controlled trial of out-patient treatments. Br J Psychiatry 2001;178:216-21.

229. Geist R, Heinmaa M, Stephens D, et al. Comparison of family therapy and family group psychoeducation in adolescents with anorexia nervosa. Can J Psychiatry 2000;45(2):173-8.

230. Robin AL, Siegel PT, Koepke T, et al. Family therapy versus individual therapy for adolescent females with anorexia nervosa. J Dev Behav Pediatr 1994;15(2):111-6.

231. Russell GF, Szmukler GI, Dare C, et al. An evaluation of family therapy in anorexia nervosa and bulimia nervosa. Arch Gen Psychiatry 1987;44(12):1047-56.

232. Hall A, Crisp AH. Brief psychotherapy in the treatment of anorexia nervosa. Outcome at one year. Br J Psychiatry 1987;151:185-91.

233. Pillay M, Crisp AH. The impact of social skills training within an established in-patient treatment programme for anorexia nervosa. Br J Psychiatry 1981;139:533-9.

234. Thien V, Thomas A, Markin D, et al. Pilot study of a graded exercise program for the treatment of anorexia nervosa. Int J Eat Disord 2000;28(1):101-6.

235. le Grange D, Eisler I, Dare C, et al. Evaluation of family treatments in adolescent anorexia nervosa: a pilot study. Int J Eat Disord 1992;12(4):347-57.

236. Robin AL, Siegel PT, Moye AW, et al. A controlled comparison of family versus individual therapy for adolescents with anorexia nervosa. J Am Acad Child Adolesc Psychiatry 1999;38(12):1482-9.

237. Robin AL, Siegel PT, Moye A. Family versus individual therapy for anorexia: impact on family conflict. Int J Eat Disord 1995;17(4):313-22.

238. Gowers S, Norton K, Halek C, et al. Outcome of outpatient psychotherapy in a random allocation treatment study of anorexia nervosa. Int J Eat Disord 1994;15(2):165-77.

239. Eisler I, Dare C, Russell G, et al. Family and individual therapy in anorexia nervosa. A 5-year follow-up. Arch Gen Psychiatry 1997;54(11):1025-30.

240. Klerman G, Weissman M, Rounsaville B, Chevron E. Interpersonal Psychotherapy of Depression. New York, NY: Basic Books, Inc.; 1984.

241. Fairburn CG. Interpersonal psychotherapy for bulimia nervosa. In: Klerman G, Weissman M, editors. New Applications of Interpersonal Psychotherapy. Washington, DC: American Psychiatric Press;1993:355-78.

242. Lock J, le Grange D, Agras W, Dare C. Treatment manual for anorexia nervosa: A family-based approach. New York: Guilford Press; 2001.

243. Gartlehner G, Hansen RA, Kahwati L et al. Drug class review on second generation antidepressants: Updated report. Chapel Hill, NC: Prepared by RTI-UNC Evidence-based Practice Center for The Agency for Healthcare Research and Quality;2005.

244. Beumont PJ, Russell JD, Touyz SW, et al. Intensive nutritional counselling in bulimia nervosa: a role for supplementation with fluoxetine? Aust N Z J Psychiatry 1997;31(4):514-24.

245. Carruba MO, Cuzzolaro M, Riva L, et al. Efficacy and tolerability of moclobemide in bulimia nervosa: a placebo-controlled trial. Int Clin Psychopharmacol 2001;16(1):27-32.

246. Faris PL, Kim SW, Meller WH, et al. Effect of decreasing afferent vagal activity with ondansetron on symptoms of bulimia nervosa: a randomised, double-blind trial. Lancet 2000;355(9206):792-7.

247. Fichter MM, Kruger R, Rief W, et al. Fluvoxamine in prevention of relapse in bulimia nervosa: effects on eating-specific psychopathology. J Clin Psychopharmacol 1996;16(1):9-18.

248. Fichter MM, Leibl K, Rief W, et al. Fluoxetine versus placebo: a double-blind study with bulimic inpatients undergoing intensive psychotherapy. Pharmacopsychiatry 1991;24(1):1-7.

249. Fluoxetine Bulimia Nervosa Collaborative Study Group. Fluoxetine in the treatment of bulimia nervosa. A multicenter, placebo-controlled, double-blind trial. Fluoxetine Bulimia Nervosa Collaborative Study Group. Arch Gen Psychiatry 1992;49(2):139-47.

250. Goldstein DJ, Wilson MG, Thompson VL, et al. Long-term fluoxetine treatment of bulimia nervosa. Fluoxetine Bulimia Nervosa Research Group. Br J Psychiatry 1995;166(5):660-6.

251. Hoopes SP, Reimherr FW, Hedges DW, et al. Treatment of bulimia nervosa with topiramate in a randomized, double-blind, placebo-controlled trial, part 1: improvement in binge and purge measures. J Clin Psychiatry 2003;64(11):1335-41.

252. Kanerva R, Rissanen A, Sarna S. Fluoxetine in the treatment of anxiety, depressive symptoms, and eating-related symptoms in bulimia nervosa. Nord J Psychiatry 1994;49(7):237-42.

253. Kennedy SH, Goldbloom DS, Ralevski E, et al. Is there a role for selective monoamine oxidase inhibitor therapy in bulimia nervosa? A placebo-controlled trial of brofaromine. J Clin Psychopharmacol 1993;13(6):415-22.

254. Romano SJ, Halmi KA, Sarkar NP, et al. A placebo-controlled study of fluoxetine in continued treatment of bulimia nervosa after successful acute fluoxetine treatment. Am J Psychiatry 2002;159(1):96-102.

255. Pope HGJr, Keck PEJr, McElroy SL, et al. A placebo-controlled study of trazodone in bulimia nervosa. J Clin Psychopharmacol 1989;9(4):254-9.

256. Sundblad C, Landen M, Eriksson T, et al. Effects of the androgen antagonist flutamide and the serotonin reuptake inhibitor citalopram in bulimia nervosa: a placebo-controlled pilot study. J Clin Psychopharmacol 2005;25(1):85-8.

257. Walsh BT, Hadigan CM, Devlin MJ, et al. Long-term outcome of antidepressant treatment for bulimia nervosa. Am J Psychiatry 1991;148(9):1206-12.

258. Goldstein DJ, Wilson MG, Ascroft RC, et al. Effectiveness of fluoxetine therapy in bulimia nervosa regardless of comorbid depression. Int J Eat Disord 1999;25(1):19-27.

259. Hedges DW, Reimherr FW, Hoopes SP, et al. Treatment of bulimia nervosa with topiramate in a randomized, double-blind, placebo-controlled trial, part 2: improvement in psychiatric measures. J Clin Psychiatry 2003;64(12):1449-54.

260. Agras WS, Rossiter EM, Arnow B, et al. Pharmacologic and cognitive-behavioral treatment for bulimia nervosa: a controlled comparison. Am J Psychiatry 1992;149(1):82-7.

261. Goldbloom DS, Olmsted M, Davis R, et al. A randomized controlled trial of fluoxetine and cognitive behavioral therapy for bulimia nervosa: short-term outcome. Behav Res Ther 1997;35(9):803-11.

262. Mitchell JE, Fletcher L, Hanson K, et al. The relative efficacy of fluoxetine and manual-based self-help in the treatment of outpatients with bulimia nervosa. J Clin Psychopharmacol 2001;21(3):298-304.

263. Mitchell JE, Halmi K, Wilson GT, et al. A randomized secondary treatment study of women with bulimia nervosa who fail to respond to CBT. Int J Eat Disord 2002;32(3):271-81.

264. Walsh BT, Wilson GT, Loeb KL, et al. Medication and psychotherapy in the treatment of bulimia nervosa. Am J Psychiatry 1997;154(4):523-31.

265. Walsh BT, Fairburn CG, Mickley D, et al. Treatment of bulimia nervosa in a primary care setting. Am J Psychiatry 2004;161(3):556-61.

266. Agras WS, Schneider JA, Arnow B, et al. Cognitive-behavioral and response-prevention treatments for bulimia nervosa. J Consult Clin Psychol 1989;57(2):215-21.

267. Fairburn CG, Jones R, Peveler RC, et al. Psychotherapy and bulimia nervosa. Longer-term effects of interpersonal psychotherapy, behavior therapy, and cognitive behavior therapy. Arch Gen Psychiatry 1993;50(6):419-28.

268. Wolk SL, Devlin MJ. Stage of change as a predictor of response to psychotherapy for bulimia nervosa. Int J Eat Disord 2001;30(1):96-100.

269. Agras WS, Walsh T, Fairburn CG, et al. A multicenter comparison of cognitive-behavioral therapy and

interpersonal psychotherapy for bulimia nervosa. Arch Gen Psychiatry 2000;57(5):459-66.

270. Bulik CM, Sullivan PF, Carter FA, et al. The role of exposure with response prevention in the cognitive-behavioural therapy for bulimia nervosa. Psychol Med 1998;28(3):611-23.

271. Bulik CM, Sullivan PF, Joyce PR, et al. Predictors of 1-year treatment outcome in bulimia nervosa. Compr Psychiatry 1998;39(4):206-14.

272. Carter FA, McIntosh VV, Joyce PR, et al. Role of exposure with response prevention in cognitive-behavioral therapy for bulimia nervosa: three-year follow-up results. Int J Eat Disord 2003;33(2):127-35.

273. Chen E, Touyz SW, Beumont PJ, et al. Comparison of group and individual cognitive-behavioral therapy for patients with bulimia nervosa. Int J Eat Disord 2003;33(3):241-54; discussion 255-6.

274. Cooper PJ, Steere J. A comparison of two psychological treatments for bulimia nervosa: implications for models of maintenance. Behav Res Ther 1995;33(8):875-85.

275. Davis R, McVey G, Heinmaa M, et al. Sequencing of cognitive-behavioral treatments for bulimia nervosa. Int J Eat Disord 1999;25(4):361-74.

276. Fairburn C, Jones R, Peveler R, et al. Three psychological treatments for bulimia nervosa. A comparative trial. Arch Gen Psychiatry 1991;48(5):463-9.

277. Fairburn C, Peveler R, Jones R, et al. Predictors of 12-month outcome in bulimia nervosa and the influence of attitudes to shape and weight. J Consult Clin Psychol 1993;61(4):696-8.

278. Garner DM, Rockert W, Davis R, et al. Comparison of cognitive-behavioral and supportive-expressive therapy for bulimia nervosa. Am J Psychiatry 1993;150(1):37-46.

279. Griffiths RA, Hadzi-Pavlovic D, Channon-Little L. A controlled evaluation of hypnobehavioural treatment for bulimia nervosa: immediate pre-post treatment effects. Eur Eat Disord Rev 1994;2(4):202-20.

280. Hsu LK, Rand W, Sullivan S, et al. Cognitive therapy, nutritional therapy and their combination in the treatment of bulimia nervosa. Psychol Med 2001;31(5):871-9.

281. Laessle RG, Beumont PJ, Butow P, et al. A comparison of nutritional management with stress management in the treatment of bulimia nervosa. Br J Psychiatry 1991;159:250-61.

282. Safer DL, Telch CF, Agras WS. Dialectical behavior therapy for bulimia nervosa. Am J Psychiatry 2001;158(4):632-4.

283. Sundgot-Borgen J, Rosenvinge JH, Bahr R, et al. The effect of exercise, cognitive therapy, and nutritional counseling in treating bulimia nervosa. Med Sci Sports Exerc 2002;34(2): 190-5.

284. Thackwray DE, Smith MC, Bodfish JW, et al. A comparison of behavioral and cognitive-behavioral interventions for bulimia nervosa. J Consult Clin Psychol 1993;61(4):639-45.

285. Treasure JL, Katzman M, Schmidt U, et al. Engagement and outcome in the treatment of bulimia nervosa: first phase of a sequential design comparing motivation enhancement therapy and cognitive behavioural therapy. Behav Res Ther 1999;37(5):405-18.

286. Ventura M, Bauer B. Empowerment of women with purging-type bulimia nervosa through nutritional rehabilitation. Eat Weight Disord 1999;4(2):55-62.

287. Wilfley DE, Agras WS, Telch CF, et al. Group cognitive-behavioral therapy and group interpersonal psychotherapy for the nonpurging bulimic individual: a controlled comparison. J Consult Clin Psychol 1993;61(2):296-305.

288. Wilson GT, Fairburn CC, Agras WS, et al. Cognitive-behavioral therapy for bulimia nervosa: time course and mechanisms of change. J Consult Clin Psychol 2002;70(2):267-74.

289. Crosby RD, Mitchell JE, Raymond N, et al. Survival analysis of response to group psychotherapy in bulimia nervosa. Int J Eat Disord 1993;13(4):359-68.

290. Bailer U, de Zwaan M, Leisch F, et al. Guided self-help versus cognitive-behavioral group therapy in the treatment of bulimia nervosa. Int J Eat Disord 2004;35(4):522-37.

291. Carter JC, Olmsted MP, Kaplan AS, et al. Self-help for bulimia nervosa: a randomized controlled trial. Am J Psychiatry 2003;160(5):973-8.

292. Durand MA, King M. Specialist treatment versus self-help for bulimia nervosa: a randomised controlled trial in general practice. Br J Gen Pract 2003;53(490):371-7.

293. Thiels C, Schmidt U, Treasure J, et al. Guided self-change for bulimia nervosa incorporating use of a self-care manual. Am J Psychiatry 1998;155(7):947-53.

294. Treasure J, Schmidt U, Troop N, et al. Sequential treatment for bulimia nervosa incorporating a self-care manual. Br J Psychiatry 1996;168(1):94-8.

295. Braun DL, Sunday SR, Fornari VM, et al. Bright light therapy decreases winter binge frequency in women with bulimia nervosa: a double-blind, placebo-controlled study. Compr Psychiatry 1999;40(6):442-8.

296. Esplen MJ, Garfinkel PE, Olmsted M, et al. A randomized controlled trial of guided imagery in bulimia nervosa. Psychol Med 1998;28(6):1347-57.

297. Mitchell JE, Agras WS, Wilson GT, et al. A trial of a relapse prevention strategy in women with bulimia nervosa who respond to cognitive-behavior therapy. Int J Eat Disord 2004;35(4):549-55.

298. Turnbull SJ, Schmidt U, Troop NA, et al. Predictors of outcome for two treatments for bulimia nervosa: short and long-term. Int J Eat Disord 1997;21(1):17-22.

299. Fichter MM, Leibl C, Kruger R, et al. Effects of fluvoxamine on depression, anxiety, and other areas of general psychopathology in bulimia nervosa. Pharmacopsychiatry 1997;30(3):85-92.

300. Agras WS, Rossiter EM, Arnow B, et al. One-year follow-up of psychosocial and pharmacologic treatments for bulimia nervosa. J Clin Psychiatry 1994;55(5):179-83.

301. Wilson GT, Loeb KL, Walsh BT, et al. Psychological versus pharmacological treatments of bulimia nervosa: predictors and processes of change. J Consult Clin Psychol 1999;67(4):451-9.

302. Fairburn CG. Overcoming Binge Eating. New York: Guilford; 1995.

303. Cooper P. Bulimia nervosa: a guide to recovery. London: Robinson; 1993.

304. Esplen M, Garfinkel PE. Guided imagery treatment to promote self-soothing in bulimia nervos: a theoretical rationale. J Psychother Pract Res 1998;7:102-18.

305. Arnold LM, McElroy SL, Hudson JI, et al. A placebo-controlled, randomized trial of fluoxetine in the treatment of binge-eating disorder. J Clin Psychiatry 2002;63(11):1028-33.

306. Hudson JI, McElroy SL, Raymond NC, et al. Fluvoxamine in the treatment of binge-eating disorder: a multicenter placebo-controlled, double-blind trial. Am J Psychiatry 1998;155(12):1756-62.

307. Pearlstein T, Spurell E, Hohlstein LA, et al. A double-blind, placebo-controlled trial of fluvoxamine in binge eating disorder: a high placebo response. Arch Women Ment Health 2003;6(2):147-51.

308. McElroy SL, Hudson JI, Malhotra S, et al. Citalopram in the treatment of binge-eating disorder: a placebo-controlled trial. J Clin Psychiatry 2003;64(7):807-13.

309. McElroy SL, Casuto LS, Nelson EB, et al. Placebo-controlled trial of sertraline in the treatment of binge eating disorder. Am J Psychiatry 2000;157(6):1004-6.

310. Laederach-Hofmann K, Graf C, Horber F, et al. Imipramine and diet counseling with psychological support in the treatment of obese binge eaters: a randomized, placebo-controlled double-blind study. Int J Eat Disord 1999;26(3):231-44.

311. McElroy SL, Arnold LM, Shapira NA, et al. Topiramate in the treatment of binge eating disorder associated with obesity: a randomized, placebo-controlled trial. Am J Psychiatry 2003;160(2):255-61.

312. Appolinario JC, Bacaltchuk J, Sichieri R, et al. A randomized, double-blind, placebo-controlled study of sibutramine in the treatment of binge-eating disorder. Arch Gen Psychiatry 2003;60(11):1109-16.

313. Stunkard A, Berkowitz R, Tanrikut C, et al. d-fenfluramine treatment of binge eating disorder. Am J Psychiatry 1996;153(11):1455-9.

314. Ricca V, Mannucci E, Mezzani B, et al. Fluoxetine and fluvoxamine combined with individual cognitive-behaviour therapy in binge eating disorder: a one-year follow-up study. Psychother Psychosom 2001;70(6):298-306.

315. Grilo CM, Masheb RM, Wilson GT. Efficacy of cognitive behavioral therapy and fluoxetine for the treatment of binge eating disorder: a randomized double-blind placebo-controlled comparison. Biol Psychiatry 2005;57(3):301-9.

316. Agras WS, Telch CF, Arnow B, et al. Weight loss, cognitive-behavioral, and desipramine treatments in binge eating disorder: an additive design. Behavior Therapy 1994;25:225-38.

317. Grilo CM, Masheb RM, Salant SL. Cognitive behavioral therapy guided self-help and orlistat for the treatment of binge eating disorder: a randomized, double-blind, placebo-controlled trial. Biol Psychiatry 2005;57(10): 1193-201.

318. Wilfley DE, Welch RR, Stein RI, et al. A randomized comparison of group cognitive-behavioral therapy and group interpersonal psychotherapy for the treatment of overweight individuals with binge-eating disorder. Arch Gen Psychiatry 2002;59(8):713-21.

319. Hilbert A, Tuschen-Caffier B. Body image interventions in cognitive-behavioural therapy of binge-eating disorder: a component analysis. Behav Res Ther 2004;42(11):1325-39.

320. Gorin A, Le Grange D, Stone A. Effectiveness of spouse involvement in cognitive behavioral therapy for binge eating disorder. Int J Eat Disord 2003;33(4):421-33.

321. Telch CF, Agras WS, Linehan MM. Dialectical behavior therapy for binge eating disorder. J Consult Clin Psychol 2001;69(6):1061-5.

322. Agras WS, Telch CF, Arnow B, et al. Does interpersonal therapy help patients with binge eating disorder who fail to respond to cognitive-behavioral therapy? J Consult Clin Psychol 1995;63(3):356-60.

323. Eldredge KL, Stewart Agras W, Arnow B, et al. The effects of extending cognitive-behavioral therapy for binge eating disorder among initial treatment nonresponders. Int J Eat Disord 1997;21(4):347-52.

324. Pendleton VR, Goodrick GK, Poston WS, et al. Exercise augments the effects of cognitive-behavioral therapy in the treatment of binge eating. Int J Eat Disord 2002;31(2):172-84.

325. Riva G, Bacchetta M, Cesa G, et al. Six-month follow-up of in-patient experiential cognitive therapy for binge eating disorders. Cyberpsychol Behav 2003;6(3):251-8.

326. Carter JC, Fairburn CG. Cognitive-behavioral self-help for binge eating disorder: a controlled effectiveness study. J Consult Clin Psychol 1998;66(4):616-23.

327. Peterson CB, Mitchell JE, Engbloom S, et al. Self-help versus therapist-led group cognitive-behavioral treatment of binge eating disorder at follow-up. Int J Eat Disord 2001;30(4):363-74.

328. Peterson CB, Mitchell JE, Engbloom S, et al. Group cognitive-behavioral treatment of binge eating disorder: a comparison of therapist-led versus self-help formats. Int J Eat Disord 1998;24(2):125-36.

329. Levine MD, Marcus MD, Moulton P. Exercise in the treatment of binge eating disorder. Int J Eat Disord 1996;19(2):171-7.

330. Riva G, Bacchetta M, Baruffi M, et al. Virtual-reality-based multidimensional therapy for the treatment of body image disturbances in binge eating disorders: a preliminary controlled study. IEEE Trans Inf Technol Biomed 2002;6(3):224-34.

331. Schork E, Eckert E, Halmi K. The relationship between psychopathology, eating disorder diagnosis, and clinical outcome at 10-year follow-up in anorexia nervosa. Compr Psychiatry 1994; 35:113-23.

332. Gowers SG, Weetman J, Shore A, et al. Impact of hospitalisation on the outcome of adolescent anorexia nervosa. Br J Psychiatry 2000;176:138-41.

333. Johnson C, Tobin DL, Dennis A. Differences in treatment outcome between borderline and nonborderline bulimics at one-year follow-up. Int J Eat Dis 1990;9(6):617-27.

334. Herzog W, Deter HC, Fiehn W, et al. Medical findings and predictors of long-term physical outcome in anorexia nervosa: a prospective, 12-year follow-up study. Psychol Med 1997;27(2):269-79.

335. Pinter O, Probst M, Vandereycken W, et al. The predictive value of body mass index for the weight evolution in anorexia nervosa. Eat Weight Disord 2004;9(3):232-5.

336. Saccomani L, Savoini M, Cirrincione M, et al. Long-term outcome of children and adolescents with anorexia nervosa: study of comorbidity. J Psychosom Res 1998;44(5):565-71.

337. Tolstrup K, Brinch M, Isager T, et al. Long-term outcome of 151 cases of anorexia nervosa. The Copenhagen Anorexia Nervosa Follow-Up Study. Acta Psychiatr Scand 1985;71(4):380-7.

338. Eckert ED, Halmi KA, Marchi P, et al. Ten-year follow-up of anorexia nervosa: clinical course and outcome. Psychol Med 1995;25(1):143-56.

339. Fichter MM, Quadflieg N. Six-year course and outcome of anorexia nervosa. Int J Eat Disord 1999;26(4):359-85.

340. Isager T, Brinch M, Kreiner S, et al. Death and relapse in anorexia nervosa: survival analysis of 151 cases. J Psychiatr Res 1985;19(2-3):515-21.

341. Strober M, Freeman R, Morrell W. The long-term course of severe anorexia nervosa in adolescents: survival analysis of recovery, relapse, and outcome predictors over 10-15 years in a prospective study. Int J Eat Disord 1997;22(4):339-60.

342. Bulik CM, Sullivan PF, Fear JL, et al. Outcome of anorexia nervosa: eating attitudes, personality, and parental bonding. Int J Eat Disord 2000;28(2):139-47.

343. Deter HC, Herzog W. Anorexia nervosa in a long-term perspective: results of the Heidelberg-Mannheim Study. Psychosom Med 1994;56(1):20-7.

344. Gillberg C, Råstam M, Gillberg IC. Anorexia nervosa: physical health and neurodevelopment at 16 and 21 years. Dev Med Child Neurol 1994;36(7):567-75.

345. Gillberg IC, Råstam M, Gillberg C. Anorexia nervosa outcome: six-year controlled longitudinal study of 51 cases including a population cohort. J Am Acad Child Adolesc Psychiatry 1994;33(5):729-39.

346. Gillberg IC, Råstam M, Gillberg C. Anorexia nervosa 6 years after onset: Part I. Personality disorders. Compr Psychiatry 1995;36(1):61-9.

347. Lee S, Chan YY, Hsu LK. The intermediate-term outcome of Chinese patients with anorexia nervosa in Hong Kong. Am J Psychiatry 2003;160(5):967-72.

348. Löwe B, Zipfel S, Buchholz C, et al. Long-term outcome of anorexia nervosa in a prospective 21-year follow-up study. Psychol Med 2001;31(5):881-90.

349. Råstam M, Gillberg C, Wentz E. Outcome of teenage-onset anorexia nervosa in a Swedish community-based sample. Eur Child Adolesc Psychiatry 2003;12 Suppl 1:I78-90.

350. Sullivan PF, Bulik CM, Fear JL, et al. Outcome of anorexia nervosa: a case-control study. Am J Psychiatry 1998;155(7):939-46.

351. Tanaka H, Kiriike N, Nagata T, et al. Outcome of severe anorexia nervosa patients receiving inpatient treatment in Japan: an 8-year follow-up study. Psychiatry Clin Neurosci 2001;55(4):389-96.

352. Wentz E, Gillberg C, Gillberg IC, et al. Ten-year follow-up of adolescent-onset anorexia nervosa: psychiatric disorders and overall functioning scales. J Child Psychol Psychiatry 2001;42(5):613-22.

353. Dancyger IF, Sunday SR, Eckert ED, et al. A comparative analysis of Minnesota Multiphasic Personality Inventory profiles of anorexia nervosa at hospital admission, discharge, and 10-year follow-up. Compr Psychiatry 1997;38(3):185-91.

354. Hebebrand J, Himmelmann GW, Herzog W, et al. Prediction of low body weight at long-term follow-up in acute anorexia nervosa by low body weight at referral. Am J Psychiatry 1997;154(4):566-9.

355. Morgan HG, Purgold J, Welbourne J. Management and outcome in anorexia nervosa. A standardized prognostic study. Br J Psychiatry 1983;143: 282-7.

356. Råstam M, Gillberg IC, Gillberg C. Anorexia nervosa 6 years after onset: Part II. Comorbid psychiatric problems. Compr Psychiatry 1995;36(1):70-6.

357. Crisp AH, Callender JS, Halek C, et al. Long-term mortality in anorexia nervosa. A 20-year follow-up of the St George's and Aberdeen cohorts. Br J Psychiatry 1992;161:104-7.

358. Strober M, Freeman R, Bower S, et al. Binge eating in anorexia nervosa predicts later onset of substance use disorder: a ten-year prospective, longitudinal follow-up of 95 adolescents. J Youth Adolesc 1996;25(4):519-32.

359. Herzog W, Schellberg D, Deter HC. First recovery in anorexia nervosa patients in the long-term course: a discrete-time survival analysis. J Consult Clin Psychol 1997;65(1):169-77.

360. Ivarsson T, Råstam M, Wentz E, et al. Depressive disorders in teenage-onset anorexia nervosa: a controlled longitudinal, partly community-based study. Compr Psychiatry 2000;41(5):398-403.

361. Wentz E, Gillberg IC, Gillberg C, et al. Ten-year follow-up of adolescent-onset anorexia nervosa: physical health and neurodevelopment. Dev Med Child Neurol 2000;42(5):328-33.

362. Nilsson EW, Gillberg C, Gillberg IC, et al. Ten-year follow-up of adolescent-onset anorexia nervosa: personality disorders. J Am Acad Child Adolesc Psychiatry 1999;38(11):1389-95.

363. Lee S, Chan YY, Kwok K, et al. Relationship between control and the intermediate term outcome of anorexia nervosa in Hong Kong. Aust N Z J Psychiatry 2005;39(3):141-5.

364. Møller-Madsen S, Nystrup J, Nielsen S. Mortality in anorexia nervosa in Denmark during the period 1970-1987. Acta Psychiatr Scand 1996;94(6):454-9.

365. Deter HC, Schellberg D, Kopp W, et al. Predictability of a favorable outcome in anorexia nervosa. Eur Psychiatry 2005;20(2):165-72.

366. Halvorsen I, Andersen A, Heyerdahl S. Good outcome of adolescent onset anorexia nervosa after systematic treatment. Intermediate to long-term follow-up of a representative county-sample. Eur Child Adolesc Psychiatry 2004;13(5):295-306.

367. Ben-Tovim DI, Walker K, Gilchrist P, et al. Outcome in patients with eating disorders: a 5-year study. Lancet 2001;357(9264):1254-7.

368. Franko DL, Keel PK, Dorer DJ, et al. What predicts suicide attempts in women with eating disorders? Psychol Med 2004;34(5):843-53.

369. Herzog DB, Dorer DJ, Keel PK, et al. Recovery and relapse in anorexia and bulimia nervosa: a 7.5-year

follow-up study. J Am Acad Child Adolesc Psychiatry 1999;38(7):829-37.

370. Herzog DB, Field AE, Keller MB, et al. Subtyping eating disorders: is it justified? J Am Acad Child Adolesc Psychiatry 1996;35(7):928-36.

371. Herzog DB, Greenwood DN, Dorer DJ, et al. Mortality in eating disorders: a descriptive study. Int J Eat Disord 2000;28(1):20-6.

372. Keel PK, Dorer DJ, Eddy KT, et al. Predictors of mortality in eating disorders. Arch Gen Psychiatry 2003;60(2):179-83.

373. Patton GC. Mortality in eating disorders. Psychol Med 1988;18(4):947-51.

374. Herzog W, Deter HC. [Long-term follow-up: methodologic aspects in the interpretation of follow-up results. A presentation exemplified by anorexia nervosa]. 40. 1994:117-27.

375. Fairburn CG, Cooper Z, Doll HA, et al. The natural course of bulimia nervosa and binge eating disorder in young women. Arch Gen Psychiatry 2000;57(7):659-65.

376. Fairburn CG, Norman PA, Welch SL, et al. A prospective study of outcome in bulimia nervosa and the long-term effects of three psychological treatments. Arch Gen Psychiatry 1995;52(4):304-12.

377. Fairburn CG, Stice E, Cooper Z, et al. Understanding persistence in bulimia nervosa: a 5-year naturalistic study. J Consult Clin Psychol 2003;71(1):103-9.

378. Fichter MM, Quadflieg N. Twelve-year course and outcome of bulimia nervosa. Psychol Med 2004;34(8):1395-406.

379. Gendall KA, Bulik CM, Joyce PR, et al. Menstrual cycle irregularity in bulimia nervosa. Associated factors and changes with treatment. J Psychosom Res 2000;49(6):409-15.

380. Herzog DB, Sacks NR, Keller MB, et al. Patterns and predictors of recovery in anorexia nervosa and bulimia nervosa. J Am Acad Child Adolesc Psychiatry 1993;32(4):835-42.

381. Jäger B, Liedtke R, Lamprecht F, et al. Social and health adjustment of bulimic women 7-9 years following therapy. Acta Psychiatr Scand 2004;110(2):138-45.

382. Keel PK, Mitchell JE, Davis TL, et al. Relationship between depression and body dissatisfaction in women diagnosed with bulimia nervosa. Int J Eat Disord 2001;30(1):48-56.

383. Keel PK, Mitchell JE, Davis TL, et al. Impact of definitions on the description and prediction of bulimia nervosa outcome. Int J Eat Disord 2000;28(4):377-86.

384. Keel PK, Mitchell JE, Miller KB, et al. Long-term outcome of bulimia nervosa. Arch Gen Psychiatry 1999;56(1):63-9.

385. Keel PK, Mitchell JE, Miller KB, et al. Predictive validity of bulimia nervosa as a diagnostic category. Am J Psychiatry 2000;157(1):136-8.

386. Stice E, Fairburn CG. Dietary and dietary-depressive subtypes of bulimia nervosa show differential symptom presentation, social impairment, comorbidity, and course of illness. J Consult Clin Psychol 2003;71(6):1090-4.

387. Fichter MM, Quadflieg N, Gnutzmann A. Binge eating disorder: treatment outcome over a 6-year course. J Psychosom Res 1998;44(3-4):385-405.

388. Wilfley DE, Friedman MA, Dounchis JZ, et al. Comorbid psychopathology in binge eating disorder: relation to eating disorder severity at baseline and following treatment. J Consult Clin Psychol 2000;68(4):641-9.

389. Busetto L, Segato G, De Luca M, et al. Weight loss and postoperative complications in morbidly obese patients with binge eating disorder treated by laparoscopic adjustable gastric banding. Obes Surg 2005;15(2):195-201.

390. Hay P, Bacaltchuk J, Claudino A, et al. Individual psychotherapy in the outpatient treatment of adults with anorexia nervosa. Cochrane Database Syst Rev 2003;(4):CD003909. DOI: 10.1002/14651858.

391. Hay P, Bacaltchuk J, Stefano S. Psychotherapy for bulimia nervosa and binging. Cochrane Database Syst Rev 2004;(3):CD000562. DOI: 10.1002/14651858.

392. Bacaltchuk J, Hay P. Antidepressants versus placebo for people with bulimia nervosa. Cochrane Database Syst Rev 2003;(4):CD003391. DOI: 10.1002/14651858.

393. Bacaltchuk J, Hay P, Trefiglio R. Antidepressants versus psychological treatments and their combination for bulimia nervosa. Cochrane Database Syst Rev 2001;4:CD003385. DOI: 10.1002/14651858.

394. Yanovski SZ, Yanovski JA. Obesity. N Engl J Med 2002;346(8):591-602.

395. Halmi KA, Agras WS, Crow S, et al. Predictors of treatment acceptance and completion in anorexia

nervosa: implications for future study designs. Arch Gen Psychiatry 2005;62(7):776-81.

396. Mokdad AH, Bowman BA, Ford ES, et al. The continuing epidemics of obesity and diabetes in the United States. J Am Med Assoc 2001;286(10):1195-200.

397. Flegal KM, Carroll MD, Ogden CL, et al. Prevalence and trends in obesity among US adults, 1999-2000. JAMA 2002;288(14):1723-7.

398. National Task Force on the Prevention and Treatment of Obesity. Dieting and the development of eating disorders in overweight and obese adults. Arch Intern Med 2000;160(17):2581-9.

399. Butryn ML, Wadden TA. Treatment of overweight in children and adolescents: does dieting increase the risk of eating disorders? Int J Eat Disord 2005;37(4):285-93.

400. Wadden TA, Foster GD, Sarwer DB et al. Dieting and the development of eating disorders in obese women: results of a randomized controlled trial. 80. 2004:560-8.

401. Neumark-Sztainer D. Can we simultaneously work toward the prevention of obesity and eating disorders in children and adolescents? Int J Eat Disord 2005;38(3):220-7.